Open-Heart Surgery Under 5

A Brief Narrative of My Journey

Kelly Libatique

ISBN: 9798559398303

www.KLVoice.com
Cover design by 100Covers
Interior design by FormattedBooks

Contents

Introduction

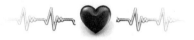

**"Take care of your body. It's the
only place you have to live."**

-Jim Rohn

As I drew closer to middle age, I started seeing a new pattern of behavior forming, a mindset and way of thinking. I began to see just how crucial it was to be deliberate about health. It started with cutting back on certain foods I enjoyed and forcing myself to get used to others I previously had not. It continued with staying more active and putting a priority on good, quality sleep at night. It was a lot of things I just didn't think about when I was younger. But in some ways, I was too late.

I once heard someone say something in a movie. It was an older, successful businessman at a retirement party who was giving some pearls to the younger guy who was going to succeed him. He made the comment, referring to his wife, "When Gloria died, all the fun went out of it." He then looked at the younger man and said, "Your wife and your health, that's the real stuff."

I was in my 20's when I saw the film, and while the remark didn't really make that big of an impression at the time, I knew I wouldn't forget it. Still though, I was going to do two things for almost the next two decades—not eat very healthy, and ignore certain health conditions I knew I should be paying more attention to.

It's not that I allowed myself to become obese or abuse drugs or anything like that. In fact, I've enjoyed good health most of my life and have stayed in decent shape. I used to run every morning, before my knees started hurting. I also participated in theatre productions that involved a lot of physical movement and dancing. I've done a lot of weight training and I enjoy juggling, including weighted balls, torches and swords. To look at me, you'd think I was fine, health-wise.

But along the way, I was overlooking a couple matters I knew were potentially serious. The first was an ongoing problem with high blood pressure. My father had it and had taken medication for years, so I figured it could be something I would have to deal with. Doctors had warned me for a long time and encouraged treatment, but I staved them off.

The second was sleep issues. I had been snoring, loudly, since I was a teenager. By the time I was in my 20's, still slender and physically active, people noticed I had a "disorder." This problem would cause me to stop breathing at night, to the point where it was almost killing me at times. I would later find out this condition is called Sleep Apnea.

But like so many things in life, I didn't do anything about any of this until I had to. The result was damage to my body that needed repair. By the time things came to fruition, I was like a 49-year-old car that had to be taken to the garage and have parts fixed and replaced.

I couldn't believe it. I was too young, too healthy, too… *something*, to have to deal with this kind of thing. But yet there I was, with only one realistic and daunting option.

I would find out later though that in addition to certain health items I'd been turning a blind eye to, there were also some preexisting conditions I was born with. None of us have any control over things like that. But in my case, the combination of what I was born with and persisting untreated problems created a perfect storm, and I ended up with two major issues that required significant medical intervention.

The first was an *ascending aortic aneurysm*. The aortic artery is the all-important hose that stems from the heart, travels up toward your head, then goes all the way down your torso to your legs, delivering freshly oxygenated blood. The aneurysm, or weakened part that was bulging out, was right where the aorta attaches to the heart.

The second problem I had was an *insufficient aortic valve*, partially related to the aneurysm. The heart has four valves that control the direction and flow of blood in and out of the heart. The final stop, before leaving the heart, is the aortic valve. Blood is supposed to go only one way, out of the heart and into the rest of the body. But since my valve was diseased and ruined, blood was "leaking" backward, back into the left ventricle in a condition called regurgitation.

To fix these problems, I needed to have one of the most invasive and dangerous surgeries performed on me—full blown open-heart surgery.

Join me on my journey from diagnosis, to testing, to surgery and continuing recovery. Everyone has their own unique set of circumstances, but if you or someone you know is in a similar situation, I hope my story both inspires and helps you prepare as you go along this voyage called life.

The Diagnosis

**"Procrastination makes easy things
hard, and hard things harder."**

—Mason Cooley

S o how did I find out about this aortic aneurism and blown valve? Hate to say it, but it was almost by accident.

Doctors have a job most couldn't do. The majority of us couldn't get through the whole med school thing to begin with. If physicians do good, they're your best friend, but if they mess up, they're your worst enemy. At least that's how it is for many. They get sued all the time for malpractice and have to pay huge insurance premiums. They're under a ton of stress and often appear overly busy.

Despite all this, most doctors I've met try to be amiable and genuinely care about their patients. But while they've spent years in school and taking tests and doing internships to ensure they're qualified, it is we, their patients, who must take charge of our own health. Assume nothing when it comes to health. Doctors are not magicians or mind readers. If there's something going on you need them to check, take the initiative and be very specific. It could save your life.

I would find out later, by the way, that the "stumbling upon" my condition story isn't all that unique and that's how many end up in cardiovascular treatment. Case in point. I'd been told for years my blood pressure was too high, but not exceptionally high. High enough to imply I may need medication *eventually*, but not anything urgent.

At doctor's offices, we learn how to hack high blood pressure numbers, to a certain degree anyway. You sit quietly and breathe deep—and I mean slow, deep, breathing. This can bring numbers down quite a bit, at least temporarily. I've done it at home too and it really does work. So when I'd go to the doctor's and get the usual blood pressure check, it would often be high at first. So they'd have me sit there and breathe. Sometimes I'd stand and rest my arm on something while they re-took the figures. Eventually, the numbers became just tolerable enough for them to send me home without insisting on any medication.

But while this technique makes the numbers prettier, they aren't exactly realistic. Do we sit around all day at work quietly deep breathing? The fact is that I had inherited high blood pressure from my father (who had taken meds for years for it) and in my case, was worsened by years of untreated sleep apnea. I'll talk in more detail of these things shortly.

But I was in denial. I didn't want to take medication. Over the years we'd all seen strange things happen to my father because of blood pressure medications. For example, sometimes he'd spontaneously fall asleep somewhere when he'd taken too much. It looked as if he was almost passing out, which in retrospect, he was. This scared me and I didn't want to depend on drugs, so over the years I'd avoided the subject.

But in the last two or three years before finally really getting a doctor to check, my blood pressure was getting increasingly worse. No matter what I did, no matter how much weight I lost or what supplements I took, it kept going higher. And I was taking a lot of supplements—vitamins B, C, D, and K, magnesium, potassium, fish oil, PQQ, turmeric and so on. All the stuff others assured me would help drop the numbers. This big pile of pills every day. I would find out later you can really overdo this stuff, especially after age 40. I was also drinking lots of green and hibiscus tea and I don't even like the taste of that stuff. To boot, a book I'd read assured me that if I switched my diet to vegetarian, my blood pressure would drop, so I even tried that.

But none of it was working. The blood pressure continued to rise.

One day I got scared when I was having a typical day at work and wandered over to the training center where they have these little desk blood pressure monitors. I put my arm in the Velcro sleeve and checked, and my systolic was 165, diastolic was 97! We also have a machine at home I'd inherited from my mother in law and after this I started regularly checking my blood pressure, especially in the morning. One morning it was like 170 over 95. And then another morning it was almost 180! Yikes. Typically, if your systolic number is 180 or higher, they check you into emergency for fear you'll have a stroke. If you don't know what those numbers mean, I go over them in the next chapter.

So I went to the doctor, again, and said look, is there anything else that can be done before I finally succumb to meds to help this blood pressure thing? I was at a point to where I was open to treatment as long as it wasn't just

3

a bandage for something more serious. He looked at the computer and said that when I came in, my blood pressure "wasn't that high," like 142 over 86 (other doctors would say this *is*, in fact, high). Doctors are accustomed to seeing high blood pressure numbers when people first walk in because many have had a busy day and are anxious about being at the doctor's office in the first place. But then I told him about how high I'd seen it lately in various times throughout the day.

He breaks out his stethoscope and this time really starts slowly going over parts of my chest, back, and even neck. In medical terminology, they call this *auscultation*, from the Latin verb auscultare, "to listen," when one listens to the internal sounds of the body. When he paused at one point, I looked up at his face and saw him frowning and shaking his head. I call this, the *uh, oh frown*, because when your doctor frowns like that, you say, 'Uh oh…'

"What's wrong?" I asked.

"I hear a heart murmur," he said.

I now know a lot about the heart. In fact, I might even be able to fool a novice that I'd at least gone to med school at one point if I start talking about the heart, arteries, veins and valves and how it all works. Heck, I could teach a class about heart murmurs. But at this point in time, while I had heard the term before, I had no idea what it was.

Think of a garden hose. If you're holding a hose while watering the shrubs in your yard, the flow of water through it sounds and feels normal, if there are no kinks or blockages. You can feel the steady, vibrating flow of liquid. But if you step on part of the hose or kink it, you both feel and hear the hiss of water trying to squeeze though the narrowed area. Same thing if you put your thumb over the end to make the water squirt harder. There are several varieties, but any abnormal sounds like that are *heart murmurs*. As the doctor is listening, he or she can hear that at least something isn't right, even if what's precisely wrong can't be identified.

In my case, there were no blockages, or "kinks in the hoses," which various tests would later confirm. But I did have what's called a *sever aortic valve regurgitation*. That's when the valve isn't working and blood flows the wrong way. But we didn't know that yet.

There are four valves a normal human is born with. These valves control the direction of the blood flow. And this is important. In simple terms, "used" blood that has been depleted of oxygen, makes its rounds throughout veins your body, and eventually ends up in the right chambers of the heart where it's pumped to the lungs to get resupplied. After acquiring more oxygen, the blood is moved to the left chambers. Its last main stop in your heart is the lower left chamber or left ventricle.

Between heartbeats, the aortic valve (sometimes called the *aortic semilunar valve*) relaxes and lets the new, fresh blood into the upper left chamber where the aortic artery is connected. The valve then closes to stop the blood from going backwards, back into the left ventricle. Then, with the next beat, off it goes up the aortic artery, first ascending to smaller carotid arteries that carry blood to your brain, and then down through your abdomen where it branches out to each of your legs in the femoral arteries. Eventually, blood will end up in the tiniest of capillaries to feed your muscles and organs. After making its rounds, veins carry the blood back to the heart to start over again.

The following simple graphic shows the body's circulatory system. The red lines are freshly oxygenated blood and the blue lines are "used" blood. The grey triangular shapes at the top are the lungs.

Graphic: Blood circulation in the body

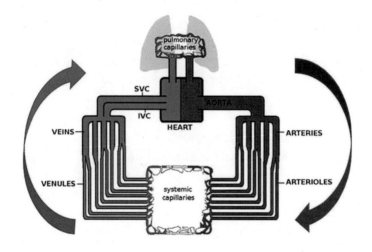

Image Source: Gccwang (Jun. 10, 2020.) In Wikipedia. Retrieved from https://en.wikipedia.org/wiki/Hemodynamics ("Circular" arrows on each side added by Kelly Libatique)

The aortic artery, starting from the heart, looks like a big candy cane in your body. The portion attached to your heart, the root section that goes up before curving over and down, is called the *ascending aorta*. After feeding the brain, it descends behind your main gut near your spine. I have a nice graphic of it in the "Ascending Aortic Root Aneurism" chapter.

It's a wonderfully engineered system that does its thing over and over, hundreds of times per hour. Adult men should be doing 60—100 heartbeats per minute and women, 60—70; this number goes up with pregnancy. This partly explains why men in general have more heart attacks—our hearts work more throughout our lifespans.

Anyway, when the doctor finally really listened to my heart, he could hear the regurgitation as blood leaked backwards, back into the left ventricle. The flaps on my aortic valve were not working correctly. To compensate for this insufficiency, my heart had been having to work harder and harder to get the same amount of blood through my body as it would if the valve was functioning properly.

Think of it this way. Say, in a normal day, your heart had to pump the equivalent of 1,500 gallons around your body to sustain it. But if you had blockages or leaky valves, your heart would have to pump hard enough to send, say, 2,000 gallons to make up the difference. And of course, any physical activity only increases the need.

If your heart is doing double duty, one of things that can happen is that it begins to thicken unnaturally. Why? Well, when you start weight training by doing curls with dumbbells, what happens? Your bicep muscles get bigger, much more so than if you did not do the exercise. It's the same with your heart, which is basically a muscle with hollow chambers inside. The more and harder it pumps, the bigger and stronger it gets.

Now, you'd think that's good right, your heart getting stronger. No…a thickened heart muscle has stiffer walls and can affect heart valves. In many people this has caused their mitral valve to become leaky. The mitral is the valve between the left atrium and the left ventricle of the heart, consisting of two tapered cusps. Thickened heart walls can also mess with the electrical conducting system of the heart which can cause abnormal heart rates or rhythms to develop, leading to cardiac arrest. All of this is *no bueno*.

Your heart beats correctly using a precise electrical sequence. It begins in the right atrium and spreads throughout the atria (the atria receives blood returning to the heart from the body, then ventricles pump blood from the heart to the body). From there, electrical impulses travel down a group of specialized fibers to all parts of the ventricles (in a human's four-chambered heart, there are two ventricles: the right which pumps blood into the pulmonary circulation to the lungs, and the left which pumps blood into the aorta). This exact route must be followed for the heart to pump properly.

What can also happen when the heart muscle is damaged, is that the heart enlarges. This is called, ready?—a *cardiomegaly* or *idiopathic dilated cardiomyopathy*. This can happen because of blocked coronary arteries and/or high blood pressure. It can also temporarily happen because of pregnancy. As the heart gets bigger, muscle cells do not increase and therefore have to work harder to keep a now larger mass going. Symptoms start with shortness of breath, swelling of one's legs, constant fatigue all the time, strange feeling heartbeats like skipped or extra beats and so on.

Eventually, you're going to have big problems, like dying of a heart attack or being severely disabled by one.

By the way, if you're wondering what the difference is between a heart attack and a cardiac arrest, I'll give you a blurb here. Buildings have both plumbing and electricity and so do our bodies. Heart attacks are plumbing problems, cardiac arrests are electrical problems.

If your coronary arteries get clogged by plaque or what have you, the areas of the heart not getting enough blood start to quit and eventually die, leading to a heart attack. But with a cardiac arrest, the heart's built-in electrical conduction system that keeps it beating at a steady pace is impaired. The causes can be high blood pressure, infections, and other things resulting in the heart not beating effectively. This happened to a coworker of mine. He was at a restaurant and felt something wrong with his heart and collapsed. He later found out that an infection from a tooth traveled down to his heart disrupting the electrical sequence and causing it to beat out of rhythm. Blood flow was effectively halted. He almost died, and would have if the cook hadn't performed *cardiopulmonary resuscitation* (chest compressions) on him.

But going back to me—at this point, all my doctor had was a heart murmur. No cause, no specific diagnosis as to what kind of murmur. Nothing would be for sure until after a whole bunch more tests. The official diagnosis would come after the echocardiogram, which I'll go into in the next couple sections. I'll also explain what exactly an aortic aneurism is and what specifically was happening to me.

But first, a little on blood pressure.

High Blood Pressure

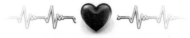

"Opportunity seldom rises with blood pressure."

—Jarod Kintz

There's been a lot more talk about high blood pressure as of late and for good reason. For a while now it's been affecting one in four Americans, but as of this writing, it's closer to one in three. It seems the western world in particular has grown increasingly stressed out over everything. America is one of the most medicated societies in the world and we're paying a huge price in terms of health care, substance abuse, addiction treatment, mental health and other problems.

Along with this stress has come hypertension, or high blood pressure. It's known as "the silent killer," because a person rarely feels symptoms. But if left untreated, can lead to all sorts of problems including blindness and kidney failure.

But it's the millions of heart attacks, heart disease and strokes high blood pressure is responsible for that many mistakenly attribute to other things like poor diet, a lack of exercise and being overweight. While all these things can contribute to and aggravate a situation, it's the high blood pressure itself that many overlook.

Again, symptoms are rare, but when it's really bad, a person might have headaches, slightly blurred vision or palpitations. As with myself, you can have it for years and not know it until your doctor one day tells you about the permanent damage it has done to your kidneys, heart, or eyeball arteries. Well okay, I had been warned it was high, but not *dangerously* high.

The only way to know if you have high blood pressure is to have it checked. And today we don't have to go to the doctor to do that as technology has made it affordable to have a small machine at your home or work where you can easily monitor it for yourself anytime. But you still should go to the doctor, of course. In fact, I'd take your home machine to the doctor's so that you can compare numbers with the more sophisticated and expensive devices the doctor has. Blood pressure machines, by the way, are called *sphygmomanometers*. Don't you just love medical terminology?

All that aside, high blood pressure runs in my family and I should have known better. My father was on medication for decades for it. A self-described "triple type-A personality," my father went through life uptight and stressed out about things. While I didn't inherit the full brunt of his "AAA" personality, I did inherit the blood pressure problem. By the way, an uptight persona doesn't cause high blood pressure, but it can augment it. My mother is the opposite and has had blood pressure so low, during checkups, doctors have asked if she was dizzy or feeling okay. She always was. Ah well, we can't choose what we inherit.

As I said, doctors have always told me my blood pressure was a little high but it didn't become anything that really concerned me until shortly before my diagnosis. And what constitutes *high* is still debatable.

So there's two numbers to be considered when you take your blood pressure. Example, you go to the doctor and get the cuff on your arm and after getting squeezed and slowly let go, the machine says your pressure is, say, 130 over 75. The machine is measuring arterial pressure and then making calculations. The force or pressure, by the way, is measured in millimeters of mercury, or mmHg.

The "upper" number, called the *systolic* pressure, represents the amount of pressure on your arteries when the heart pumps, or with each beat of your heart. In other words, when the left ventricle contracts. The "lower" number is the *diastolic* pressure and it represents the pressure in your arteries between heartbeats, or when your heart is at rest.

The systolic reading is the one most strongly linked with heart disease, but both values are important with regards to your health. A high systolic reading typically means an increased risk of heart attacks and heart disease more, whereas a high diastolic reading has been linked with a higher risk for disease involving the aorta, the problem I had.

Arteries have stretchy walls, by the way, compared to veins, because they need to handle the most pressure. The heart is powerful. If you cut a main artery, blood can squirt as far as 30 feet in the air. This is why coronary angiograms are a bit risky, and I go over that procedure in a later chapter.

It used to be that if your blood pressure was below 140 over 90, you were considered fine. Now they are saying it should be below 120 over 80. These numbers change with age, by the way. If you're young, like below age 20, it should definitely be well below 120 over 80. But as a person ages, arteries typically get stiffer, so blood pressure goes up. By the time you get to my age, roughly 139 over 88 is still considered okay by many but again, the standards are still changing.

My blood pressure has never been that low anyway. Typically, I'd go to the doctor's and when I first walked in, it'd be like 147 over 90. So they'd have me sit quietly and breathe deep for a good five minutes, then do it again and have my arm resting on something level with my shoulder. Sometimes they'd have me stand. This usually brought the numbers down to around 140 over 80-something and they'd be happy with that and send me home. This went on for years, so I figured nothing was wrong, or at least that bad.

Blood pressure is a strange thing and when modern medicine practitioners are honest, they really don't know what causes it. We do know what can agitate it—a high sodium diet, smoking, alcohol abuse, obesity and so on. Correcting or quitting these things can bring it back down to its default levels. But what sets the bar in one's body, as it were, in different individuals is a mystery. Non-Hispanic, black people, for example, have much higher rates of hypertension than other groups and its unknown why. It's also mysterious why and how the kidneys play a role. If you get a kidney transplant, for example, your blood pressure will eventually change to match or come close to the blood pressure of the donor from whom you acquired the kidney. Very mystifying.

The next image is of a small blood pressure machine at my place of work. Notice the number 111 next to "SYS" (systolic) and the 76 next to "DIA" (diastolic). If you ever take a reading and the numbers are this low, you're in good shape, at least with regards to blood pressure.

Photo: Blood pressure machine

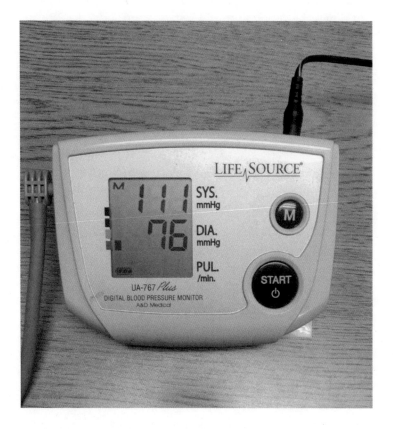

Image Source: Kelly Libatique (n.d.). No copyright.

I mention all this because my high blood pressure did damage to what doctors think was an already damaged aortic artery root in me. As you now know, one's aorta is the main hose that takes freshly oxygenated blood and sends it on down the pipeline to the rest of your body. It's kind of important. In my case, the aortic root, right where it connects to the heart, was already oversized and the more it stretched, the worse my valve was getting on top of that. Or at least that was one theory.

It can be thought of this way. If you have a double-door, like French Doors, and the door frame was flexible and you stretched it apart, what would happen to the doors? They would not close properly and leave a gap. The other theory involved numerous ways heart valves can become diseased and don't open or close properly for a bunch of reasons. You can be born with certain conditions, or high blood pressure and other things that can weaken valve performance. Under some conditions, the leaflets, or "flaps" of the valve, can become stiff and calcified. Whatever the case, high blood pressure was making a bad situation in me worse and now, downright dangerous.

The takeaway from all this is, if you suspect you have high blood pressure or if it runs in your family, have it checked. It really doesn't take much. Especially as you age, you need to get it checked more regularly. There's a lot of older, even slender people going around with high blood pressure. You may be lucky and not need any meds—just a few changes in your lifestyle.

Remember, you can be skinny and have high blood pressure, or be overweight and have normal numbers. I've known heavy smokers who have low blood pressure numbers. You can be a quiet, introverted person that everyone who knows you would describe as calm and peaceful, but have high blood pressure. You can have a "AAA" uptight personality like my father and have normal readings. You get the idea.

Franklin Roosevelt—"FDR"—the 32nd president of the U.S., had extremely high blood pressure, like in the 260 over 150 kind of range. He wasn't someone described as hyper, nervous or tense all the time. It's a wonder he never had a stroke in front of the cameras. He ended up with congestive heart disease though and died abruptly of a cerebral hemorrhage. He's a classic case of untreated high blood pressure. His doctors knew about it, but they just didn't have the meds we have today to ease symptoms.

The bottom line is that if you do have it and leave it untreated, there will be consequences, the degree of which only depends on the level of pressure and the amount of time it was untreated. I finally got mine treated, but damage had already been done.

Sleep Apnea

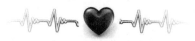

**"Sleep is the golden chain that binds
our bodies and health together."**

—Thomas Dekker

I've been a pretty healthy person most of my life. I attribute much of that to my genetic makeup which consists of a variety of DNA from around the globe. I have grandparents with roots from Germany, England, Ireland and Spain. I also have a grandparent from Asia and on that side, there is also Spanish, Chinese, Basque French and even Aborigine. Like dogs, when you mix breeds, the stronger, dominant traits tend to supersede the weaker and you typically end up with creatures that have less problems than purebreds. *Woof...*

This has been the case for me. I've enjoyed correction-free eye sight and hearing, have had to endure almost zero dental work, and always had a good metabolism. I get very few colds and flus, and haven't had to battle obesity. I've never had any cancer, diabetes, thyroid or join disorders. Bottom line, I've had it pretty good when it comes to health.

Except for a couple things. Big things. Besides high blood pressure, my biggest disorder is obstructive sleep apnea. And like high blood pressure, this condition has gotten a lot more attention in the last few years as some high profile individuals have actually died from it or from complications caused by it: James Gandolfini, John Candy, Carrie Fisher, to name a couple. This condition is for real, and I almost died from it myself.

In simple terms, sleep apnea is where you stop breathing when you fall asleep. By medical definition, you have sleep apnea when you "frequently stop breathing for 10 seconds or longer during sleep." I used to frequently stop for a lot longer than that. It happens mostly at night, but falling asleep anywhere at any time causes it.

What happens is your throat closes up and your airway is stopped. Think of it this way. Remember when they still made plastic straws with the paper wrapper? My kids, when they were little, in restaurants, would rip off one end and blow the other off like a missile at each other, scoring if it hit someone in the eye. Well, if you take one of those paper straw wrappers and dip one end in water then try to suck air through the dry end, what happens? The wet end clamps together causing a blockage.

This is what happens during sleep apnea. Just as you're really drifting off into a deep sleep, somewhere between stage three and four, the kind that produces dreams. It's when all your muscles are relaxing and getting disconnected from the brain. As your diaphragm is expanding to open your lungs, they suck in air like fireplace billows. But then the top of your throat relaxes and closes like the wet end of the straw wrapper. This shuts your windpipe tight, and I mean literally airtight. This happens over and over, all night, resulting in you never going into REM (rapid eye movement) or stage four sleep. You instead spend the night bouncing back and forth mostly between stage one and three, snoring and choking yourself awake just as you're going into the sleep you need. You can lay in bed for eight hours this way and wake up feeling miserable, like you still need a nap—because you do.

Many think sleep apnea only happens to overweight people, but I've had this condition since my early 20's when I was pretty slender. It's some kind of physical defect in the throat I was born with. Even when I was younger and skinnier, I've always had a double-chin when I look down, and this extra mass in my throat has, in part, led to my sleep apnea. But even slender looking people with no double-chin can have this problem.

I remember times in the middle of the night I'd suddenly get jolted awake, gasping desperately for air, my body covered in sweat and my heart feeling like it was thumping a million beats per minute. I found out later that due to my sleep apnea, I would cease breathing for such long periods of time, my heart would stop and I'd actually lie there in a state of being clinically dead. As a last-ditch effort to save itself, my brain would send an electrical charge to my heart, similar to what a defibrillator does, and jump start it. I can remember feeling the shock and pain travel quickly from my head to my chest and it was scary and startling. This happened to me several times during my younger years. And I can remember horrifying dreams that sometimes accompanied these events. One in particular was of me drowning. I'd be under water struggling frantically to breathe and I'd believe I was actually about to die until something woke me and I could suck air in again. Yeah, real fun stuff.

The significance of all this was not made known to me until years later when I was almost 40. And like many things in life, it came unexpectedly, in my case, from an allergy doctor.

I've always had horrendous seasonal allergies and for the most part just took a lot of over-the-counter stuff to deal with it. Finally, one year, it was so bad, I saw an allergy specialist who started asking me if I snore at night and things like that. Of course, my sleep apnea and other subjects came up, and he sent me home with a device that measures my blood oxygen saturation throughout the night—a fingertip pulse oximeter of some type.

When I returned and gave the oximeter back, the doctor was shocked. He said my blood oxygen was dropping to 40% at night. I was literally being choked and gagged all night by my own throat. Imagine a sinister and sadistic person or evil spirit sitting on your bed watching you try to sleep and every time you really started drifting off, would take hold of your throat and strangle you. The doctor said if I don't do something about this and get treatment, I was going to ruin my heart and become a "cardiac cripple" for the rest of my life. People with this condition can't go anywhere without an oxygen tank on wheels and tubes sticking out of their noses. This seemed persuasive and got my attention, and with the urging of my wife and others, I decided to go to my regular doctor and get referred for a sleep study.

I should mention here that sleep apnea can also lead to other fun stuff like diabetes, depression, an abnormal heart rhythm, heart failure, coronary artery disease and stroke. It's serious stuff. Sleep deprivation is so devastating to both the mind and body, it has been used as a form of torture. But that's another story. On with the sleep study.

In a nutshell, a sleep study is where you spend the night in a clinic with wires all over your body, similar to when you get an EKG. I will never forget that night. They do their best to make the room up like a regular bedroom, complete with homey but pleasant décor and such. But it's still a laboratory with a machine full of wires on the nightstand and an infrared camera mounted on the wall facing the bed.

It was nearly impossible to fall sleep and I know I irritated the staff by asking them several times to unplug me so I could use the restroom. But finally, somehow, I managed to drift off, but only for a couple hours. I'd actually more or less passed out from exhaustion rather than fell asleep. But two hours was enough. The sleep doctor who looked at the results the next morning said he didn't have to "see the whole movie, just a snippet." And what he saw made him quickly draw the conclusion that I have "severe, *life-threatening* obstructive sleep apnea."

This explained a lot of things. It explained why, for years, no matter how long I had lain in bed, I was tired and felt like I wanted a nap. It explained why, if I had to drive for more than 15 or 20 minutes, I would start falling asleep behind the wheel. I could describe several incidents where I almost got into serious accidents because of this. It explained why at my work, where I was behind a computer most of the day, I would constantly be dozing off. I would get caught snoring in my cubical, so I learned how to nap with my forehead resting in my palms because when gravity was pulling my neck forward instead of toward the back of my throat (like when lying on my back) there was less chance of choking and snoring. If there was a meeting, I could not concentrate because I was drifting off. After dinner in the evenings when my wife wanted a little conversation, I would be falling asleep on her. I would be on vacation and trying to enjoy a ride around some place or in a concert or show, but I'd be nodding off the whole time. People would comment on the bags under my eyes and dark circles around them and ask me if I was okay. Everywhere and under all circumstances, I was tired and wanted to make up on sleep.

How could you live with this for so long?, you ask. Well, like many things in life, you can become fatalistic and think that's just the way you are. I thought I was just a tired person in general. I'd lived with fatigue for so long, I didn't know any other way to feel and had nothing to compare it to.

After the official diagnosis, I talked to my doctor about treatment options. Some people wear this mouthpiece thing at night that holds the jaw forward so there's less chance of the throat closing up. Some use this as a solution for bad snoring alone. But my doctor didn't think this would help as my apnea was too severe. There is also surgery which removes the palatine uvula and part of the soft palate that is believed to be responsible for what happens during sleep apnea. But the doctor I was seeing was anti-surgery in his philosophy. He invited me to get other opinions on the matter if I wanted, but stated that he's seen surgery do either no good or make matters even worse. In his opinion, surgery wasn't worth the risks. In the end I took his advice and he became my primary sleep doctor for years. He still would be if my insurance provider hadn't changed.

Ultimately, I was prescribed a CPAP machine (continuous positive air pressure). It's essentially a fancy air pump. You wear a mask over your nose that pushes air down your throat all night and keeps the airway open. Some have to use a larger mask that also covers their mouth and even their whole face, but I've only used the nasal kind.

They've come a long way with CPAP technology. The machines are remarkably quiet and the headgear and masks are very comfortable. They're also "smart" nowadays by capturing your breathing patterns and then easing up on the air pressure as you're exhaling and then increasing it again as you inhale.

But it's still something strapped to your face at night. The first night you try to sleep with a CPAP is quite frustrating. You can feel it pressed to you, feel the air blowing in, hear the whisper of the machine and delicate hiss of air from the top of the mask. And you keep having to adjust the tension of the straps. If the straps are too lose, the mask leaks air on your face; too tight and it starts to hurt. Like anything new, it just takes some getting used to it. I was tempted to give up as many have, but I persisted and eventually I did get to sleep.

The next image is a photo of me wearing my CPAP mask.

Photo: CPAP machine

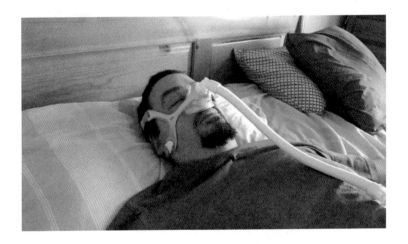

Image source: Kelly Libatique (n.d.). No copyright.

Eventually, after a struggle, I got through my first night with a CPAP. I looked at the clock and was astonished that I had slept steadily for six or seven hours with no interruptions. I felt so refreshed, I was "glowing," for lack of a better word. I hadn't had that kind of deep, sustained sleep in literally years.

I had so much energy, I didn't know what to do with it. I wanted to run around the block. I wanted to go outside and do a couple hours of yard work. I was actually reinvigorated for once instead of still feeling blah. It was a miracle and I've been using the CPAP ever since— almost nine years as of this writing. Some give up using it after awhile, but not me. I tell people like I'm telling you now, it saved my life. Plain and simple. I can't imagine sleeping without it.

The drawback is that when I travel, the CPAP goes with me. It's not a big machine, but enough to be an annoyance in terms of luggage space and such. At airports I have to take it out and show the security agents. At hotels, I have to get the part of the bed that has the best nightstand where I can setup the machine.

It makes vacations interesting too. When my kids were younger, they wanted to go camping, but that was a problem for me because I needed electricity. Nowadays they have better, smaller, portable CPAP machines that run on battery, but not then. The solution was places like KOA camps where there's a cabin with plugs next to the bed. Or at Yosemite National Park, for example, they have these tent cabins with electric outlets. Sometimes I get frustrated, but I keep reminding myself that there's worse things to live with like chronic pain or an impairment that makes you less mobile. Like most people, I've learned to do what I have to.

Another drawback is that I typically have to take a sleep aid like doxylamine and I often supplement this with melatonin. The fact of the matter is, even after all these years, unless I'm really exhausted and ready to pass out tired, the mask is still distracting. I don't like depending on pills for anything, but the older I've gotten, the more I've come to appreciate a good night's sleep. When I was in my 20's going to college, I could spend all week getting almost no sleep while I wrote papers and studied for tests. I thought nothing of it. But by the time I was almost 50, one night of no sleep can ruin several days.

So why do I bring up all this about sleep apnea? Because sleep apnea not only leads to some of the nasty stuff I mentioned earlier, but increased high blood pressure. And high blood pressure can lead to problems like damaged heart valves or further damaging an aortic aneurism or whatever else you've got going on. Remember, I went for years with untreated apnea. Two and a half decades of making my heart struggle all night, every night, had done damage that I wasn't aware of. And like so many other things, you just don't know until the damage is done.

The takeaway here is that if you have sleep apnea, or even if you just snore really loud at night, get it looked at while you're still young and haven't done any permanent damage to your body. If you're already approaching midlife as I was, or older, it's never too late to get treatment—until it kills you. Trust me, you'll appreciate any improvement, especially if you've lived with certain symptoms for a long time.

Ascending Aortic Root Aneurism

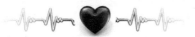

**"A thumping heart is your body's way
of saying THANK YOU."**

—Unknown

The ascending aortic root aneurism wouldn't get diagnosed until after the echocardiogram and MRI, but I'll go ahead and talk about it now. Like many who get diagnosed with something serious, I got to work doing some research to find out what I was facing. In some ways, doing all this investigating is a form of masochism, because the more you read, the more you feel like you've got all the additional symptoms and problems you're gathering information about. It gets scarier by the day. You've probably heard this happens to medical students—they call it "Medical students' disease," or "intern's syndrome." I can believe it happens a lot, even though I'll never formally study medicine at this point.

The aorta is the largest artery that carries freshly oxygenated blood to the rest of your body. It first ascends upward toward your head, where the smaller carotid arteries take blood to the brain, then curves downward behind your gut and near the spine. In pictures it looks like a big candy cane. Once near your hips, it branches out to the legs in the femoral arteries.

One of the best animated videos and explanations of the blood flow through the heart can be found on a video called "Blood Flow through the Heart in 2 MINUTES," published by Neural Academy and can be found at this URL if you want to check it out: https://www.youtube.com/watch?v=jBt5jZSWhMI

The next graphic shows the different parts of the aorta.

Graphic: Aorta segments

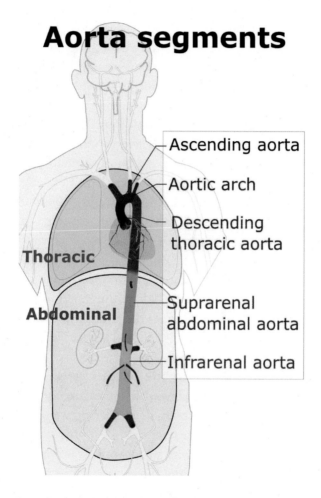

Aorta segments

- Ascending aorta
- Aortic arch
- Descending thoracic aorta
- Thoracic
- Abdominal
- Suprarenal abdominal aorta
- Infrarenal aorta

Image Source: In Wikipedia. User: Mikael Häggström, using source image by Edoarado, CC BY-SA 3.0 <https://creativecommons. org/licenses/by-sa/3.0>, via Wikimedia Commons

The *aortic root* is part of the ascending aorta and is the section of pipe directly connected to your heart. If it fails, your brain and body no longer get blood and oxygen and you die pretty fast. If it ruptures because of an aneurism, you'll die a painful death of internal bleeding fairly quickly. I was told chances of survival are roughly 50/50 if that happens, and that's if they can get you to an emergency room quickly.

A normal adult's aorta is only supposed to be two to three centimeters in diameter, give or take a bit depending on one's overall size. When a bulge starts forming that becomes one and half times greater than its average size, it's an aneurism. Think of it like a water balloon or garden hose that has a weak spot and that area starts to bulge outward because of the internal pressure. Maybe you've seen this happen to a tire on your car. Eventually it will burst, right? Or, in the case of your aorta, there's also an occurrence called a *dissection* where the innermost layer of it allows blood to flow between the layers of the aortic wall, forcing the layers apart. This can lead to a slower and uglier death of a stroke or organ failure. Pleasant stuff...

When an aneurism is still under a certain diameter, there's a chance you can avoid invasive surgery and keep it at bay by diet, proper exercise, and losing weight. And if you've got high blood pressure that won't go away, medication. The unfortunate facts are, aneurisms are irreversible, won't heal on their own, and typically continue to worsen.

There's a risk chart regarding surgery they're still perfecting, but it's getting more accurate. You see, any surgery, particularly the open-heart variety, is a dodgy undertaking—people die on the operating table or get heart attacks or strokes during or right after it which cause permanent damage or death. So it's avoided, if possible. But once an aneurism or a blockage or whatever the case is threatening a person with more risk of doing nothing than the risks of getting cut open like a fish, it's time to go under the surgeon's knife. It's the old justification principle that salesmen use to get customers to shell out—you convince them that the risks of doing nothing outweigh the costs and logistics and whatever else of buying what they're selling. In my case, I didn't need a hard sell.

Current statistics, by the way, vary. Bear in mind that the following numbers apply more to those who are older or already weakened from other illnesses. For example, once you're 85 years or older, mortality increases significantly. But here are some general numbers. For coronary bypasses, 1 to 3% don't survive the operation. For aortic valve replacement, like what I was facing, it goes up to 3 to 5%; mitral valve surgery is even slightly higher. Between 2 and almost 5% have strokes during or after surgery and of those, 60% had strokes directly after the operation; 4 in 1,000 or .4% of patients have heart attacks related to the surgery.

These numbers are creepy when you consider they are human lives—grandparents, moms, dads, even kids. But try to see it this way: if you were gambling at a casino and those were your odds of losing, you'd get rich fast. In other words, because medical science has gotten so good, the odds lean heavily in your favor.

Here's how it broke down for my condition, specifically. When an aneurism is discovered anywhere on one's aorta, they start gathering intel about your family history. Do you have any relatives that have had aneurisms, burst aortas, or dissections? Is there any diabetes or other illnesses like lose joints or retinas and things of that nature that needs to be added to the equation? Because if so, the risk chart changes and if it's your aortic root that's the problem, somewhere between 4.5 and 5 cm, they're going to tell you surgery is inevitable and you'd better start the process of preparing.

In my case, no one in my family has ever had any of those things. As I've said, I've had it pretty good with health and had no preexisting conditions. So in my case, the risk of having a burst aneurism or dissection starts getting really bad right around the 5.5 cm mark, and the possibility of things going south by doing nothing, outweighs the risks involved with open-heart surgery.

By the time I was diagnosed, my lower *descending aorta* looked okay, but my *ascending aorta* starting from the root, was 5.9 cm! Hence, the ticking time bomb and impending doom lurking behind my sternum. In fact, my cardiologist was surprised I didn't have any ongoing symptoms like chest pain or tightness, shortness of breath or swollen legs or arms. There were times I sometimes felt a little short of breath, like when under stress or after a long day, but nothing that ever really bothered me.

Nonetheless, there it was—undeniable images from both an echocardiogram and an MRI, which I'll go over shortly. This was mid-September when I was hearing this and my surgeon said that if I had wanted to wait "until next year" to fix this, he'd get very nervous for me. He told me flat out, I can either get elective surgery, or I'd be rushed in anyway in a four-alarm wagon. That seemed persuasive to me. Honestly, between how bad my case was and the COVID pandemic right around the corner, it was by God's grace that all this came to light when it did.

And thus began a series of tests to prep me for one of the biggest events in my life…

The Echocardiogram

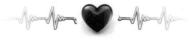

**"Medicine is a science of uncertainty
and an art of probability."**

—William Osler

I marvel at today's technology. If you went back 150 years, people would drop dead in their late 30's or early 40's and no one had any idea why. It was normal. Explains why people were getting married and having kids at teenagers—like a Mayfly, one just didn't have a lot time to live life.

But today we can look under skin, inside blood, bones, veins, even inside the very trillions of cells that make up our body. With this knowledge, we can see not only what's happening, but what may or *will* happen down the road and take preventative action.

So, the next step after the doctor heard my heart murmur was an echocardiogram. You'll often hear doctors refer to it as just an "echo." This device works like the sonograms they use to look at babies developing in the womb. It's painless, non-invasive, and doesn't do any harm (like radiation can) because it uses only high-frequency/ultrasound sound waves to produce images. The echocardiogram is engineered to look at the frequencies emitted specifically by the human heart.

For the procedure, I was taken into a large room that had a bed with a small table on rollers next to it. Mounted on the table was a large computer monitor and beneath that a control panel with a big rollerball and a bunch of different keys and knobs.

I was asked to take off my shirt and lie on the bed on my left side. The lights were then turned off, leaving the monitor as the only source of illumination. It created an interesting atmosphere, but more eerie than anything else because of why I was there.

The technician, after hitting a few keys, grabbed a tube and a wand of some sort (it's actually called a *transducer*), attached by wire to the machine, and squeezed this goopy gel onto the end from the tube. The end of the wand was semi-soft and slightly rounded; this was then inserted into a receptacle on the table which apparently heated it and the gel on it.

After a minute, the tech took the wand out and placed it on my chest. It was indeed warm, almost hot to the touch. But I guess that's a lot better than cold.

The images came up on the screen right away. I can see why they use the gel—the wand has to be moved around quite a bit, slid a quarter-inch this way and that, and aimed at different angles to get the right images. But there on the screen was my heart pulsating away. The image was grainy, a silver-white on a black background, but otherwise pretty detailed.

Eventually my aortic valve was found and I watched it open and close on the screen, over and over in a rhythmic beauty, like a little "door" opening and slamming shut. The door looked like it was struggling a bit, though. Seeing it was pretty amazing, knowing that this happens all day, every day, 5,000 per hour. Wow...

Then the sound was turned up. You could hear the swishing and swirling of blood as it travelled in and out of heart chambers and then up the aorta. I guess I was also hearing that murmur I was told about, but my ears weren't trained to know the difference between my heart sounds and a normal, healthy one where there was no regurgitation.

The whole procedure ended up being about an hour, most of it spent on my left side but a few minutes on my back. Also, an RN came in at one point and took over for a few minutes when the technician said she wasn't able to find something. At the end of it, the RN said that she'd "found your murmur," but didn't go into details.

When it was over, I didn't feel like hanging around to ask questions. So I just said thank you, wiped the goop off, threw my shirt on and got out of there.

On the next page is a still from one of the dozens of short videos of my two echocardiograms. Note that the image does it no justice. When you see it live and animated with sound, it's amazing. You can see the flaps (also called cusps or leaflets) of your heart valves opening and closing. The colors on the right side shows the deoxygenated (blue) and freshly oxygenated blood (red) as it moves around the different chambers of the heart.

Image: My echocardiogram

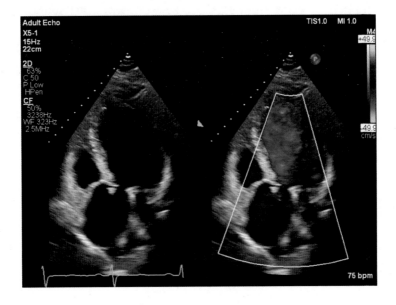

Image source: Kelly Libatique (n.d.). No copyright.

The results were sent to my doctor and the next thing I knew I was getting messages that I had a "severe aortic valve insufficiency." Apparently, my aortic valve was only 60% sufficient and the rest was leakage back into the left ventricle. My poor heart was having to work overtime to make up for this and I'd been unaware for years. They were also suspecting an aneurism. It makes you wonder how many people out there are living with things like this, totally unbeknownst to them.

The implications were enormous. Was I really going to need surgery to fix this? The reality wasn't sinking in yet. But a call from my doctor did make some things come to light. I like my doctor, he speaks fluent Spanish and Portuguese and his English has a slight accent. As a result, he doesn't mince words and goes straight to the point. He informed me that I'd probably need surgery and added, matter of fact-like, that it was a procedure that had a "low mortality rate," so I shouldn't worry.

What?

A cold feeling washed over me. I knew the answer, but had to ask. "In your opinion, will something happen in the next five years if nothing is done?"

"Definitely, in my opinion, you will have something happen within five years," he said.

Note that at this point, only the regurgitating valve was for certain. Although they were suspecting it, the full sureness of the aneurism would not be known until after the MRI. Had we known, my doctor may have said something will happen in five *weeks* instead of five years. I would have to get started educating myself about all this.

Next stop, the MRI.

Medication

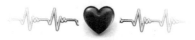

"Dear Stress, we need to break up…"

—Unknown

Before I talk about the MRI, a quick blurb on medication. Yes, I finally gave in. It took me until the ripe age of 49 and after lots of warnings. But I succumbed. I capitulated. I caved. I started taking meds for my high blood pressure.

I guess with a stubborn person like I can be, it took seeing my heart valve flapping away to tell me there were some delicate parts in my body that had been damaged or were being further damaged by high blood pressure. It took understanding that if some things didn't change, I really could end up dying while standing in line at the grocery store, clutching my chest and grimacing in pain while people captured the whole thing on their cell phones. The way things are today, someone might even livestream it on their favorite social media site. Or worse, I could be driving on the freeway when that happened. If I were an airplane pilot, there'd be a lot more at stake.

Bear in mind, I'd never taken meds for anything before. I was too healthy for that, after all. But because of the now official diagnosis of a valve regurgitation and probably of an aortic aneurism, my doctor ordered me to start taking medication. He said we need to keep your systolic number below 130 at a minimum.

There are lots of blood pressure medications out there, but they fall into several main categories. There's the diuretics which reduce fluid and sodium in the system. There's the beta blockers which act directly on the heart to reduce the rate of heartbeat and force of pumping. There's the ACE inhibitors which help keep blood vessels open by inhibiting the angiotensin-converting enzyme. And there's four or five other categories. My doctor put me on a certain beta blocker.

Beta blockers work by blocking the effects of epinephrine, which is a hormone most of us know as adrenaline. When you take beta blockers, your heart beats slower and with less force, thereby not only reducing blood pressure, but overall blood volume.

Did it work for me? Absolutely, quickly in fact. I was quite surprised at how effective it was. If I were to pick a daily average, I'd say my systolic number was routinely getting to be between 145 and 165. Those numbers represent times when I'd first hop out of bed or in the middle of the day when I'd be having a typical day at work. It quickly started averaging below 130 throughout the day which is almost the goal. And often now, months later, especially toward the evening, it's getting below 120. My diastolic number was usually between 80 and 90; it's now always below 80. And I'm not taking much, only 25 mg twice a day.

Side effects? Yes, some but not that bad. People who are active and like to run or play sports often complain that beta blockers slow them down, but I don't do much of that sort of thing anymore. I'm supposed to take it with food, but if I don't take it with a full glass of water the side effects are worse. The problem here is that I'm also not supposed to drink a lot when eating. So a good compromise is taking it with a full glass of water about 20 minutes before or after eating.

Side effects for me sometimes include a little dizziness. This is especially true for the morning dose. If I take it with only a sip of water I feel this a lot more. But again, I don't feel this much at all if I take it with a full glass.

The other main side effect is sleepiness. Not that it acts as a sleep aid, like doxylamine—more like, you feel you just don't quite have the same energy. Not having the same energy makes a person sit around more which by its nature induces a sleepy feeling. To mitigate this, I deliberately get up and walk during the day.

I also sometimes experienced cold hands in the beginning. I had read that some feel both cold hands and feet, but I usually felt no difference in my feet. I like to take long morning walks when it's still cool. At certain times, during those walks, I've definitely felt like my hands were colder than they'd normally be before I started taking this drug. After a few months though, this symptom went away.

Oh, and as a little side note—when it comes to sleeping, magnesium works wonderfully. I usually take one with the melatonin. Magnesium orotate, in particular, is what many people use as a supplement for high blood pressure. Magnesium is a naturally occurring mineral and it relaxes muscles and is good for calming nerves. I've met sleep experts who keep some on the nightstand in case they wake up in the middle of the night; magnesium helps them go back to sleep.

There are long-term side effects of beta blockers that many have reported. Real fun stuff including fatigue, weakness, dry mouth and eyes, dry skin, diarrhea, nausea and vomiting. I've not experienced any of that and goodness knows, I'd rather not. In the beginning, I figured I would be able to ween myself off this stuff in time, but after everything I know now about blood pressure, I don't think that will be possible.

The takeaway here is, we have things today when comes to medication that may help you, even if just temporarily. I get the whole anti-big pharma stuff and I can't do a lot of preaching here. I resisted for years. I get it that we have way too many prescriptions out there and that many if not most drug companies are far more into profit than people. And there's often dreadful side effects to some of these drugs that we're not warned about.

Plus, we've been trained like clapping seals to look for a pill for the solution to just about anything. Western doctors are coached to prescribe this stuff; ask them about natural remedies or herbs and you'll probably be told they've not been trained in that area, which is true. So be very honest with your doctor and express your concerns. In the end, there may be a small amount of something that will help extend your life and not damage something or create further damage in your body.

The MRI

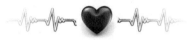

"The science of today is the technology of tomorrow."

—Edward Teller

M
any people have had a Magnetic Resonance Imaging, or MRI done for a variety of reasons and already know all about them. They are also known as 'nuclear magnetic resonance imaging,' but there's no dangerous, ionizing radiation involved. This section here is more for those who've not yet had the experience. It's not as bad as you might think, unless, of course, you're truly claustrophobic.

There is wonderfully detailed information out there about how MRI machines work, so I won't get too much into it here. I couldn't explain it that well anyway. But in a very simple nutshell, the human body is mostly water and water molecules contain hydrogen nuclei, or protons. An MRI machine's magnet can force these protons to align their angular momentum, or "spin" to a magnetic field (protons don't actually physically spin, this is a term referring to the moving forces holding protons together). The magnetic field applied by an MRI scanner is about a thousand times the strength of a typical refrigerator magnet. This sounds scary, but you don't feel it and it doesn't hurt you. When the magnetic field is turned off, the protons gradually return to their normal spin in a process called *precession*. Precession produces a radio signal that can be measured by receivers in the scanner and made into an image. Yeah, the people who figure this stuff out are good.

By the time the MRI is finished, your skin may as well be completely transparent. I used to be into aquariums, kept them for years, and it made me think of fish like the glass catfish or the Indian glassy fish. Their skin is, for all intents and purposes, invisible, and you can see every bone and organ in them. There are other fish that have see-thru skin like jellyfish and certain species of frogs and even octopus. But that's what an MRI does—it "sees" inside of you as if your skin weren't there.

A co-worker of mine had had three MRIs for his knees and back by the time I was schedule for mine, so I got an earful from him as to what to expect. But the MRI experience is different for everyone depending on their target. The target for me was smack dab in the middle of my chest.

The radiology department in hospitals tends to be in the lowest parts of the building, maybe because of the huge equipment, or maybe because there's less disturbance for the magnetic, sound and other waves the equipment utilizes. I don't know. But I can tell you it's already an odd feeling taking the elevator to the basement where you know the morgue is typically kept as well. I'm a real glass-half-full thinker, as you can see.

I'd scheduled my MRI on a Sunday evening and was the only one in line. I got there a good 30 minutes beforehand and was taken right in, about 15 minutes early, which rarely happens. A tech came out to get me, and on the way, asked the usual security/safety questions: my full name, date of birth, reason I was there and so on. He then punched a code into a keypad on the thick, heavy door and we entered a cool, dark, laboratory setting.

I'd prepared by wearing only sweatpants and a t-shirt, but they made me change into the standard aqua-green, draw string and pull-over hospital garb anyway. I was able to at least keep my underwear on which preserved a certain amount of dignity. As I'm going in, I was asked if I had any metal whatsoever on or in my body—implants, hearing aids, tooth fillings, anything. I said no (this would change after surgery). I'd even remembered to leave my wedding ring at home.

After changing and putting slip resistant socks over my own, I was escorted into an adjacent room where a giant tan colored machine sat that proudly bared the General Electric logo. I was asked if I'd been warned about an IV they had to use on me during the test. I had not. But I'd been poked for blood draws so many times over the years, especially recently, that it was no big deal. Apparently, to get a really good look at the aorta, they need to feed a dye of some kind ("gadolinium contrast media") into you that gives even clearer images of the various tubes going to and from your heart.

As I got on the bed, it occurred to me that in most pictures I'd seen of people getting MRI's, they go in headfirst. But I was going to go in feet first. If they were going to get images of my chest, I'd have to be inserted all the way into that thing. I could have asked questions, but I instead kept my mouth shut and let the professionals do their thing.

"Are you claustrophobic?" I was asked. I said I was not, though I wasn't 100% certain at that moment. What would they have done if I'd said yes? I didn't ask, but I'm sure they have sedatives to relax those who'd otherwise freak out. "Are you able to lie on your back?" I was asked. Sure, no problem.

The technician couldn't find a vein on my left arm which they try first, so he moved the equipment to my right arm and found one. I was asked to lie down on a bed that was attached to the machine and had what looked like fresh linen and pillowcases. I hoped they were fresh anyway. There were two other techs who helped me get settled in, a quiet, young guy in his 20's and a nice woman in maybe her mid-30's.

As I looked past the foot of the bed at the opening of the massive machine, I wondered if it was big enough to squeeze in my 200-pound body. Larger and heavier people than myself get this procedure done all the time so I figured I'd be okay. We've all seen movie depictions of people getting MRIs and the inside didn't look as small as what I was about to experience.

One of the techs, the nice lady, then put something on my chest and Velcro-ed it down tight. She informed me it was so they could get a better look at my chest. Okay, fine. I couldn't tell what it was and didn't bother asking. It was rectangular and weighed maybe two pounds, but the point is that I now felt really constricted.

"Can you breathe okay?" I was asked. I said yes even though I was a bit uncomfortable. I just wanted to get this over with.

Now I was asked to put my arms and hands up behind and over my head, the kind of thing you'd do if you were surrendering to someone. I was told to just relax and that a voice from the machine would tell me when to inhale, hold my breath, then relax and so on.

Just obey *The Voice*.

The nice lady produced two ear plugs which she pinched and then inserted into my ears. Then another tech put a small squeeze ball attached to a cord into my left hand and said if I have any problems, to just squeeze. *In other words*, I thought, *if I panicked.*

Lying flat on my back with my arms in that position with a contraption strapped to my chest was most uncomfortable. In my younger years I used to do a lot of weight lifting, the good'ol days when I didn't worry about things like exploding aortic arteries. The result is that my arms and chest don't have the flexibility that most have, I'm guessing. So when I lie flat on my back with my arms above me like that, I feel really tight and stretched. Combine that with some strange medical device strapped to my chest as I'm about to be inserted into a hole, and it's not something I'd do for the heck of it.

A motor hummed to life and began moving the bed into the artificial fissure of the giant machine. It moved nice and slow and it was just like a scene from a SciFi flick where someone is going in for some experiment. As I moved further into the machine's mouth and the opening came over my head, I was surprised at how close it was to my face. I'm staring up at the inside of this thing feeling nose to nose with the surface and the embedded narrow lights. In retrospect, it wasn't really that close, but it appeared that way. I felt like I was trapped inside a prop used for an engine scene in Star Trek. If I'd sneezed, I'd have gotten the inner shell in front of my face wet. The lights built into the round, interior sides at least make you feel like you haven't been buried alive. I appreciated that. Still though, I was truly helpless at this point.

A great horror movie scene would be someone in this position who, just as the entrance to the hole goes over their vision, all the lights go out in both the machine and the whole room and there's nothing but silence as you cry out for help. Yeah, I think of stuff like that. I guess feeling vulnerable and helpless describes a lot of hospital experiences.

The next photo is similar to what my General Electric MRI machine looked like.

Photo: MRI machine

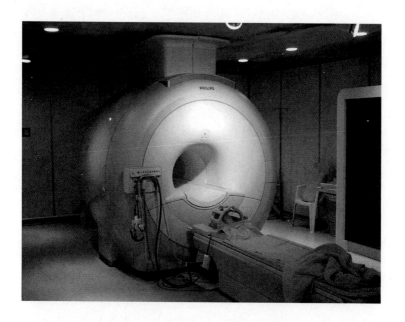

The coworker I mentioned earlier got headphones during his MRIs, wherever he'd had them. They even gave him a choice of music to listen to—rock, jazz, classical and so on. I would have chosen classical, but all I had was cheap, foam earplugs. And they didn't do that great a job.

Once the process starts, the inside of an MRI machine is loud. Not loud enough to actually hurt your ears, but enough to be a bit unpleasant. What's happening is that inside the oversized walls of the tube you're in, there are large magnets spinning around at frightening speeds. There's some great videos of this online if you want to have a look.

You first hear a series of loud clicks and knocks followed by pulsating sounds of varying frequencies. And sure enough, a computerized female voice came on and gently commanded me: "Now inhale and hold your breath." I obliged and had to wait a few seconds. Another series of pulsating sounds, these increasing with speed and rhythm. After a few seconds, "Now relax," the voice said. This routine repeated itself several times.

During this process, the bed would move slightly forward or backward, I am assuming to get the best possible position to view my innards. This went on for what seemed like quite a while. I kept trying to close my eyes and think of something else to take me away, but the noise and such made it impossible. I really wished I'd had the music option.

Finally, after what apparently was only about 10 or 12 minutes (it felt much longer), the tech's voice on speakers somewhere and said, "One more test; we'll be done in about 5 minutes." Okay, cool.

A few more clicks and beeps and then at last I heard someone say, "We're done," the nice lady I think, and the bed hummed and moved slowly back out of the tube. It was a bigger relief to have the Velcro straps undone and that thing off my chest than it was to get extracted from the tube.

While someone removed my IV, I took my earplugs out and one of the techs took them from me. I said thanks and a young male voice said, "For sure," and I was reminded how youthful he was and how dated I was starting to feel. At his age, I probably would have thought MRIs were only for "old people," and here I was.

As I walked out, I saw the main tech at a computer going over the images he'd just taken. I was tempted to walk over and ask questions, but he looked busy and concentrating hard on something. It was late on a Sunday evening and I was pretty sure I was their last patient of the day and they wanted to get out of there as much as I did. They'd taken me in early, after all. So I left him alone and exited the security door.

All in all, the whole experience was less than 30 minutes from clothes change to change and I had yet another life experience story to tell someone, sometime, just like I'm doing now.

If you ever have to get an MRI for whatever reason, know that many do, including me (not just old people), and here I am doing fine and telling you about it. Just be honest though—if you can't stand the thought of being stuck in a cramped, noisy, artificial hole for a few minutes, you need to tell someone before it starts.

In the next chapter, I will show you one of the stills from this session.

The Surgeon and my gamble

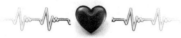

"Truth, like surgery, may hurt, but it cures."

—Han Suyin

S o before anything like a date for surgery is even suggested, you need to have an initial consultation with a cardiac surgeon. Which is a good thing. You do this to discuss options—yes there are limited options. If you're lucky, they'll tell you a less invasive surgery is available for your situation (like a transcatheter procedure). If you're even luckier, surgery may not even be necessary. The above two mentioned weren't any of *my* options.

I had my consultation in the city of Vallejo, CA. I had a choice of where the surgery would be performed: San Francisco or Santa Clara. One of the San Francisco surgeons made a trip to a Vallejo office once a week, so I took advantage of that as it's a less demanding commute from where I lived. If I was told surgery would be needed (and I had a bad feeling it was), I'd already chosen San Francisco as the location because my wife has family there and that'd make it easier for her to hang out in the area.

We met, shook hands, exchanged the usual formalities. His first name was Daniel, so for this narrative, I'll just call him "Dr. Dan." He had, of course, looked at all my test results and with a combination of both authoritative sternness and appalling casualness, informed me straightaway that I was going to need the most invasive and risky of open-heart surgery.

Don't get me wrong. Dr. Dan was a nice guy, calm, matter of fact, professional. But I was just another patient and I could tell he'd given this spiel a thousand times. Still though, I didn't feel rushed. He was there to listen and answer all my questions and concerns. If he was feigning patience and genuine sympathy for my fears, he was doing a pretty good job.

Now, I'd done my research and came prepared with questions. Why couldn't I do the transcatheter procedure I mentioned a moment ago? If you don't know, the transcatheter procedure is where they don't have to open your chest up at all. They go in through a main artery near your groin (femoral), then run a line up to your heart and replace the aortic valve that way.

Mick Jagger had the transcatheter done—for you who were born past maybe 1980, he's the singer for The Rolling Stones. When Robin Williams had his coronary angiogram in preparation for valve replacement, they went in through his femoral artery. He later joked, "Who knew that the way to man's heart was through his groin? Women are like, we've always known that…"

Nope, not an option for me. That procedure is only for aortic stenosis, where a valve is narrower than it's supposed to be, not larger like mine. With this procedure, they stick a new valve *inside* of a bad valve, not actually replace the original valve. Besides, I also needed a piece of my aortic artery (the root) replaced which is not possible without the traditional open-heart surgery. Not yet anyway.

But all my questions were made moot when the good doctor brought up a very detailed image from the MRI. Again, I marveled at today's technological capabilities. There on the screen was a perfectly clear picture of my insides, starting from about the jawline down to one of my kidneys. You could even rotate the image around and look at it from all angles; it reminded me of when Keanu Reeves was leaning back and dodging bullets in *The Matrix*. They could have done my whole body, of course, but the focus was my chest.

My aorta was a bit scary looking. As I've said, a normal adult's aorta is about 3 cm in diameter, on average. And mine, starting from the crest of the "candy cane" and on down to my kidneys looked pretty normal. Dr. Dan said my kidneys looked fine as well, by the way, which was a relief because my dad's had started to fail a few months before he died.

People get aneurisms on different parts of the aorta; you can get them down near your stomach, for example (on the "descending" part). But mine was right where the aorta attaches to the heart, the root, the "ascending" portion that goes up toward the head before curving back down the body.

And it looked ugly.

It appeared as if an otherwise perfectly fine aorta had been stepped on or crushed near the heart and then swelled up into something awful and injured. I now have forever burned in my memory what an artery that's been ballooned to almost 6 cm looks like. And you might too if you look at the image. It's actually more of the moment I won't forget, sitting there in shock in the quiet office looking at it for the first time with a surgeon.

I'd compare the aneurism, in simple visual terms, to a white, deformed upper piece of a carrot. And right where it attached to the heart, was a wrinkled opening where inside, my pitiful aortic valve was struggling fiercely, and quite futilely, to hold back blood from leaking backward.

Take a look at the next image and bear in mind that the swollen part is supposed to be no bigger than the slenderer parts.

MRI Image: My ascending aortic aneurism

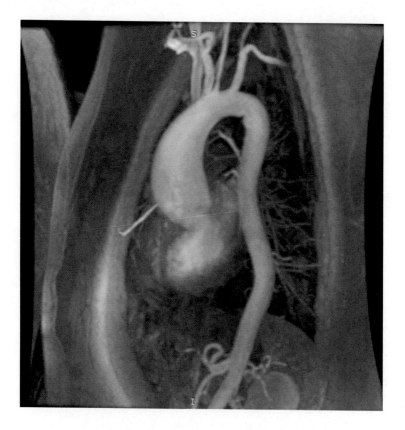

Image source: Kelly Libatique (n.d.). No copyright.

Needless to say, I was in trouble. I couldn't believe I'd been living with this for almost 50 years. Or perhaps I hadn't. Perhaps this had come about slowly, or quickly, recently. Perhaps an injury had caused it. Dr. Dan and others who'd looked couldn't tell. I racked my brain for any major impact to the chest I'd had over the years and couldn't think of any. No big car accidents or anything like that. I did do some martial arts in my younger years, but was never kicked or punched hard in the chest.

The closest I'd come to a chest injury was a couple months prior to this when I was with my 15-year-old son in San Luis Obispo at the famous Oceanic Dunes of Pismo Beach. We were in a dune buggy going too fast over some small hills and caught air off the top of one, colliding into the adjacent hill. It hurt and I got a cervical neck sprain as well as some bruises from the seatbelt. My torso hit the seatbelt hard, but that could not have been the cause of something like this.

Due to the severity of my condition, Dr. Dan thought it was hereditary, probably something I had been born with, and was really questioning me about family members who may have had anything like this. I could think of no one. I do have heart attacks in my family, but not until they were in their late 70's or early 80's. But like usual, when I tell doctors that, they don't make a big deal out of it. I guess because if you make it to that age, you've outlasted the average life expectancy anyway.

But as far as aneurisms or bad valves go, I honestly know of no one in my family who's had anything like it. Perhaps someone had, but either had never been checked for it specifically, or the technology did not yet exist. Whatever the causes, here I was at only age 49 looking at these pictures.

So…what are my options? Well, starting with the enlarged section of the aorta, this would have to get replaced.

"Replaced with what?" I asked. "Where does the material come from?"

I knew that during coronary bypass surgery, they harvest arteries from either a person's arms or legs. That way, since they come from the same body, they shouldn't be rejected. But those are small, averaging only 3 to 4 millimeters in diameter. Nothing like an aorta, which is a huge garden hose by comparison.

This, the doctor told me, again with an almost scandalously nonchalant tone, they "pull off the shelf." I envisioned a mechanic's shop with different kinds and sizes of tires and tubes hanging from the wall, which actually wasn't far from the truth. It's made of a woven polymer, like Dacron, he explained. A rubbery material similar to the stuff raincoats are made out of. And they have all different sizes—ones for a tiny person, the size of a child, to one "that would fit Shaquille O'Neal." His words, not mine.

The second problem was my aortic valve. There was a "slight chance" this could be repaired and saved once the section of aorta was swapped with the piece of Michelin Man (those are my words). But please don't count on this, I was told. Most likely, my valve would have to be replaced as well.

Okay, but replaced with what? Well, there were more choices now, *off the shelf*, and my surgeon was already heavily learning toward one. Thanks to all my own research, I actually knew 90% of what he told me about valves at that point, but I just let him talk and be the expert.

So with valve replacement, you get to choose between a synthetic or tissue valve. Both have upsides and downsides. Let's start with synthetic valves.

Artificial or mechanical valves are still commonly called "metal valves" even though the ones today don't have metal anymore. The first ones that go all the way back to the 1950's were a "caged ball" style, where a tiny steel ball, trapped in a tiny steel cage, was sewn into one's artery. The ball would get pushed to the top of the cage to let blood through when the heart pumped and then get sucked back into the hole to plug it up when the heart relaxed to stop the blood that tried to flow back. Only 57% of patients who received this kind of valve survived the first five years.

A few years later, a tilting disc style valve was invented. Same idea—the opening had a disc that swiveled from the center like the inside of a water spigot to let blood in, then swiveled back again to stop up the hole.

Today they are made of pyrolytic carbon and contain no metal at all. Most mechanical heart valves are bileaflet, meaning they have two carbon "leaflets" or flaps that open and shut like little doors to control the blood flow to a single direction. And it's this kind of valve Dr. Dan thought I should get.

By the way, of the heart's four valves - the tricuspid, pulmonary, mitral, and aortic—only the mitral valve has two leaflets, or "cusps," which is why it's sometimes referred to as the *bicuspid valve*. The rest, in a normal person with no defects, have three. Unbeknownst to anyone at this point, I actually had been born with a defect in my aortic valve, which I will discuss in later chapters.

Now let's talk about a tissue valve. A tissue valve is either harvested from a pig's heart (porcine) or fashioned from the sac surrounding the heart of a cow (bovine). These are also commonly called *bioprosthetic* valves. These tissues are treated and neutralized so that one's body will not reject them. Some tissue valves are mounted on a frame or stent, while others are stentless and used directly.

A pig's anatomy, as you may know, very closely resembles a human's in many ways. As a result, pigs have been used in some of the most hideous of medical experiments. They are used, for example, to train military medics how to plug holes and stop bleeding on the battlefield. They are also used for burned skin experiments. Ugh…But that's another story.

Pigs used for heart valves are typically the same ones slaughtered for food, so if you're a bacon or ham fan, you've no doubt eaten the meat of an animal whose heart valve ended up in a human.

Put the following address into your web browser to see a short, looped video clip (animated gif) of a pig's valve opening and closing with the beat of its heart. You can clearly see the three leaflets as they open and close:

https://upload.wikimedia.org/wikipedia/commons/d/d2/Aortic_valve.gif

The next image shows the inside of a heart, depicting the flow of blood through the various valves, veins and arteries.

Image: A heart's valves, arteries, and veins

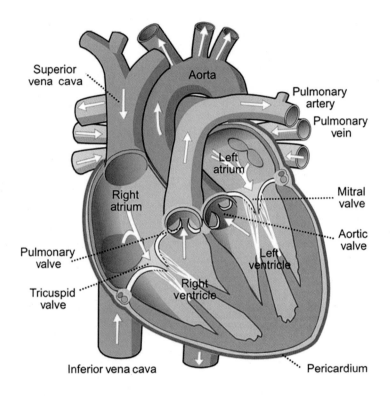

Image Source in Wikipedia: By Wapcaplet – Own work, CC BY-SA 3.0,
https://commons.wikimedia.org/w/index.php?curid=830253

The advantages and disadvantages of each type of valve vary considerably. With the mechanical valve, the advantage is that it is much more durable and can typically last 30 to 40 years without breaking down. In other words, "for life," since most people have this done in their post midlife years.

The disadvantage—and this is huge—is that the smooth surface of the flaps attracts one's body's own blood clotting or coagulating mechanism. It is, after all, artificial and the body considers it invasive. This is significant because clotting not only messes up the function of the valve, but can be deadly when later, pieces of those blood clots break off and clog up other veins, or travel to the brain and cause a stroke, an occurrence called a *thrombosis*. You may have heard the term *pulmonary thrombosis*, a potentially fatal condition where blood clots get stuck in the blood vessels of the lungs.

To mitigate the clotting problem, a person with a mechanical valve must take anti-coagulant drugs for life. These are often referred to as blood thinners even though the real function isn't *thinning* the blood, but rather to hinder blood clotting. And it's a delicate balance that has to be maintained. You have to take these drugs very precisely on just the right days and have your blood checked often—first daily, then weekly, then every 30 days. If you get out of balance and your blood gets too "thin," it will clot very little or not at all and the slightest injury could cause you to bleed to death. There's also other fun stuff like spontaneous bruising or one day dropping from a brain bleed stroke. On the other hand, if you let your balance go the other way, the clots start forming on the valve and even elsewhere where they shouldn't.

Although there are different ones now, the main anti-coagulant drug that's been in use for years and is considered the gold standard is called Warfarin or more commonly, Coumadin. It's actually been around since the 1950's. It messes with your liver to trick it into not producing as much vitamin K which is needed to cause blood clotting.

Coumadin has other fun-filled implications as well. Side effects of this drug are hardening arteries, particularly as you get older, and an increase in Alzheimer's and dementia. This drug can also make your skin look terrible with black or blue or rash like symptoms; women are more prone to this than men. Most don't have these problems in any extreme sense though.

Now, the disadvantages of tissue valves.

Since the valve is actual tissue, or flesh, you don't need to worry about clotting. Usually, one still needs to take a baby aspirin or other small amount of aspirin to keep the blood a little 'thinner' than normal, but typically, no anti-coagulating drugs are needed unless you have other conditions like a propensity for *deep venous thrombosis* or *pulmonary embolisms* that require it.

Sounds great, right? But the big drawback is that tissue valves wear out faster, particularly in younger patients. Anyone under 60 is considered young for a tissue valve. If you put one in a 20-year old, for example, they've been known to conk out in just five years. For someone my age at the time—49—it may last ten to 15 years, if I'm lucky.

This is all typically speaking of course, nothing for sure. I read one article by a cardio surgeon who happened to be against mechanical valves due to the failures and risks. He boasted that if he installed a tissue valve in you, you'd not have to worry about it wearing down, ever. Pretty bold claim that most surgeons and cardiologists don't make.

So why was my surgeon practically insisting, or acting as if the decision were already made, for me to have the mechanical valve? Simple, he didn't want to see me having to come back in ten years or less and have my chest re-opened to get another replacement. And goodness knows I didn't want that either. Surgeries on top of previous surgeries are always more dangerous. He also didn't make a big deal about Coumadin, acting as if it's effortless to use it. It's been around a long time, lots of people use it and even monitor themselves from home now, I was told. This was all true, but I don't care how long it's been around—to me that drug is still a big deal.

All that said, my decision was already pretty much made, but I'd tell him later. That decision was to roll the dice and go with a tissue valve. Here's why.

Anti-coagulant drugs scare me. My grandmother was on Coumadin for something many years ago and almost died from internal bleeding. Our bodies are brilliantly designed to know when and where to make blood clots. When we were kids and fell and scraped an elbow or knee, we took it for granted that "scabs" formed over the cut or wound to stop the bleeding. Our bodies just do that, right? It *knows* when and where it's injured.

There's actually a very complicated process that causes clotting to happen. In simple terms, platelets—tiny fragments in your blood—get triggered by a combination of things when a blood vessel is damaged. Platelets stick to the walls in the damaged area and each other, changing shape to form a stopper that fills in a cut, tear, or hole to obstruct the bleeding. One of the key dependencies of all this is one's liver's production of vitamin K. It's an amazing process and one so complex, it's a wonder it works as effectively as it does. Because when it doesn't work as it should, it's deadly. Sometimes this happens to people because of a liver disease or they damage their livers with years of alcohol abuse.

Imagine if blood clotted where it wasn't supposed to and blocked arteries and veins? Imagine if your blood didn't clot at all? Some people have to live with conditions like this for various reasons and terrible things can happen like blood clots impeding arteries and veins. Or, as I've mentioned, clots break off and get stuck in the lungs (*pulmonary embolism*) or go up to the brain and cause strokes. And again, you can bleed to death from even a small injury.

What Coumadin does specifically is that is messes with your liver's ability to produce vitamin K. It tricks it into producing less than it normally would. The implications are big. If you don't take enough, your liver will still produce enough vitamin K to clot your blood sufficiently to impair your mechanical valve. If you take too much, the opposite happens and a small injury, bruise, or damaged blood vessel anywhere in or on your body could be fatal.

There are other implications. If, say, on the week or month you have your blood checked, you'd been eating a spinach and kale salad or some other green, leafy source of vitamin K daily, you'd have to continue eating that same portion each day once the level of Coumadin is established. If you added another source of vitamin K—asparagus, avocado, etcetera—that would mess up your balance. And this should go without saying, but that vitamin K or K2 supplement someone on a YouTube video told you to take? Throw it away.

Same with alcohol which does the opposite—it "thins" the blood more. If you were having a glass of wine each night, once your Coumadin levels are set, you must stick with that routine. Any deviation could be problematic. The six-pack you enjoy on Friday night after no drinking the rest of the week? Forget it.

I realize that monitoring technology is far superior today and there are even small units people can use at home, similar to how diabetics self-monitor their blood-sugar levels; none of this was available to my grandmother. Still though, the idea of doing this tight-wire balancing act over a crocodile pit while juggling flaming torches with my blood didn't jive with me. And even if the balance is perfect, you're still prone to bruising and bleeding much more than a person who does not take Coumadin.

Additionally, you have to carry a card around with you in case you're injured and hope paramedics or doctors see it so they'll know how to handle you differently. Certainly, if I were an athlete or someone who regularly did activities which made me more susceptible to trauma and injuries, it would be a no brainer. In my case, I just want to avoid the whole complicated addition to life.

*Disclaimer: please don't let my anti-Coumadin rant dissuade you from your physician's advice. This is only my personal opinion; I'm not playing doctor here. If you need it to save or prolong your life, by all means, do what you need to do.

The next graphic image shows what my mechanical bileaflet valve looks like.

Graphic: Mechanical bileaflet heart valve

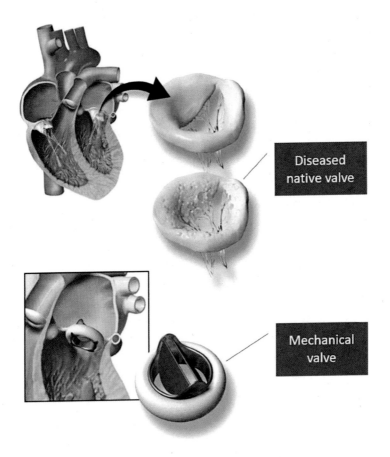

*Image source: Blausen.com staff (2014). In Wikipedia.
"Medical gallery of Blausen Medical 2014".
WikiJournal of Medicine 1 (2). DOI:10.15347/
wjm/2014.010. ISSN 2002-4436. - Own work
("Diseased native valve" and "Mechanical valve"
labels added by Kelly Libatique)*

So my decision of getting a tissue valve led to the possibility of more surgery down the road if it wears out before my expiration date. But I was banking on a couple things. The first is my generally good health. I had a good, long talk with my cardiologist a few weeks before lying down under the bright lights and sharp instruments. I really drilled him as to why tissue valves wear out the way they do, in some cases pretty quickly.

What really makes a difference is a person's overall health and other preexisting conditions. I am not overweight, do not have diabetes and eat fairly healthy. I don't smoke, I move a lot and my cholesterol has been good. In fact, when they did a rundown of bloodwork on me, they found literally nothing out of the ordinary—my electrolytes, magnesium, potassium, sodium, aldosterone, all good, and no problems with my thyroids. And I wasn't on any other medications save for the beta blockers I'd recently started taking. My two big issues have been sleep apnea and high blood pressure; the former I've been treating for years, and the latter I'd recently gotten under control. With all this going for me, there's a good chance my bioprosthetic valve would last longer than what's typical.

The second thing I was banking on is that technology is getting better all the time. They can do things via a transcatheter procedure that was unheard of just a few years ago. They fix valves without the invasive surgery all the time now. I figure if my tissue valve breaks down in, say, 15 years, the option will be there to remedy things without cutting and sawing into me again. There's even talk of sending nanobots into people's bodies to make repairs like this.

I know, I could be wrong. It was a gamble. And honestly, do any of us know if we'll be alive ten or 15 years from now anyway? Car crashes kill people all the time. Crossing the street or taking a bath is statistically more dangerous than flying across the country. Either way, I would have been rolling a lot of dice with everything I have to go through. Life forced me into this craps shoot, I'd like to think I have some semblance of control on how things go and how I live day to day until my time is up.

As we neared the end of the hour, Dr. Dan asked me if I'd been to the dentist lately. It'd been at least a couple years, I told him, maybe three. I don't see the dentist often because I've had great teeth. Well, he said, we need you to go to the dentist to have your mouth examined for infections. If anything needed doing, now was the time, *before* surgery.

I'd heard years ago that one's mouth is about the dirtiest part of the body, yes, *the* dirtiest, and apparently, bacteria and other things from one's mouth can be dangerous, even deadly, when it came to surgery. Dr. Dan went on to say that dentists tell their patients all the time that things that need fixing can be done at a later time, months, sometimes years later. This, he said, made no sense to him. If something needs to be done, why wait? So go and get checked, and if there's any impending work, *ensure the dentist gives you antibiotics*, I was warned. Okay, I said. I'd add seeing the dentist to my list of to-dos.

As we wrapped up the conversation, I told him briefly about an uncle of mine, by marriage, who had open-heart surgery about ten years prior to this and it didn't turn out well. He'd been a smoker for decades which may have contributed to his situation, I'm not sure. But he became one of the 5 to 10% of those who have a stroke during the operation. What I was told was that a tiny blood clot formed during the surgery and went to his brain. I've heard the heart and lung machine can sometimes cause this. And it was a bad stroke, a severely compromising one.

My uncle survived, but spent a couple months in the hospital curled up in the fetal position or rolling around babbling incoherently. I visited him a couple weeks after this and it was so sad. He did not recognize me and started crying, apologizing. He clearly comprehended that there were many things about him mentally and physically that were not right, but didn't understand what was going on. I did my best to be comforting, but really, what do you say?

My uncle did begin to slowly recover and all we could do was hope. Fast forward to today and he's almost 90% blind, walks with a bad limp and cane, and his mind never quite recovered. He doesn't remember a lot and often says odd and random things that make no sense. Essentially, his life was hijacked. He had been a kind, quiet, gentle person, easy to talk to and be around, very skilled with mechanics and building things. I didn't know anyone who disliked him. It really makes you wonder.

Fortunately, my uncle's children were already grown, and his son lived with him for years to take care of him because he can't function safely on his own. Later, his daughter and her husband took over. Today, his VA insurance is gone so the family does their best to care for him. He's going to need lots of help for the rest of his life.

As I told Dr. Dan about my uncle, he just nodded with a concerned frown and said, it happens, but only to a small percentage. He went on to say that he wished he could give me a guarantee, but that there was none. The facts were, I could have a stroke or heart attack from this and yes, some people don't survive at all. I appreciated his honesty and wondered to myself how anyone could become a surgeon.

How do you go out to the waiting room and tell anxious children, siblings, parents, whoever, that their loved one didn't make it through? It takes a very special kind of personality to not take things like that home and be able to start over again the next day.

I read somewhere that as of this writing, the average surgeon's salary is a little over $250,000 per year, although I'm sure that varies depending on where you live and what kind of seniority and experience you have. Not bad money, but it comes with a price. A 2012 survey said that a little over *half* of all physicians regretted their career choice and would not choose medicine again. That's huge.

My particular surgeon had been doing this nearly 30 years as of this writing and had no malpractice suits or disciplinary action against him (yeah, I did the research). I also didn't get the impression he regretted his chosen profession. But still, I was going to find out if I ended up being one of the reasons many other surgeons would have rather done something else with their lives.

As I end this chapter, I'm not going to lie. I went home and cried that night. It started as an odd feeling welling up inside and by the time it had filled me, I knew I had to cry, and hard. I cried out of self-pity and for my life potentially getting cut short. I cried that my family may lose me so soon. I cried for all the things I shouldn't have said and done to others; I cried for the things I *should* have said and done. I cried for what had happened to my uncle. I cried because we only have one life to live and I'd spent of lot of it uptight and not very happy with myself. I resolved that if I survived this, I'd try to be more productive with my borrowed time and do more of the things I enjoy.

The Coronary Angiogram

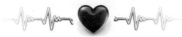

**"Science is beginning to catch up
with global health problems."**

—William Foege

One of the many tests that had to be done prior to surgery was a procedure called an *angiogram*. The official name for it is *Coronary Angiogram*, but cardiologist and surgeons will often call it a 'catheterization procedure' or just a 'cath procedure.' It's all the same thing. Due to the potential complications, they wait to do this until after the non-invasive stuff like the echocardiogram and the MRI.

Recall that arteries carry oxygenated blood from the heart to parts of your body; veins carry "used" blood back. In the case of your heart, there are small arteries called *coronary arteries* that are used to supply the heart itself with blood and oxygen. The heart is a muscle and an organ, and like all muscles and organs it needs its own supply of everything that blood contains. So when blood gets pumped out of the aorta, there are two small coronary arteries, a right and a left, that branch out of the aortic root right above the aortic valve. These arteries fork out along the heart like little tree branches, supplying the heart with the blood it just pumped.

People with lousy diets or unlucky genetics, or those who've ruined themselves with smoking and whatnot, can end up with blockages in those little branches. Once blocked, blood flow past that point is stopped and the part of the heart that was depending on it is starved. Like any organ, the parts that no longer get blood first quit, then start dying. The heart will do it's best to continue keeping you alive by forcing extra work on the parts that are still getting fed. But eventually they wear out, and along comes a visit from Heart and cousin Attack.

So when you hear about people getting coronary bypass surgery, what's happening is, the blocked arteries are too damaged to repair, so surgeons create detours. It's the same as when the freeway is blocked due to an accident or whatever; traffic gets directed around it via another route.

To create those bypasses, doctors will harvest veins from one's legs or arms. This way your body shouldn't reject them. The new veins are sewn into good parts of the upper coronary arteries, or the aortic root itself, above the blockages, and then routed around the blockages and attached.

The next page shows a graphic of the heart and coronary arteries—the red, narrowing tree root looking lines at the bottom. Notice that they start right above the aortic valve, one to the left and one to the right before branching down.

Graphic: Coronary arteries

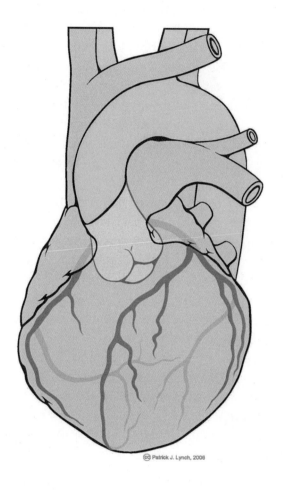

Image Source: Lynch, Patrick J. (Jul. 12, 2020.) In Wikipedia. Retrieved from https://commons.wikimedia.org/wiki/File:Coronary.pdf

With all that said, they didn't think blocked arteries were a problem for me, or so they thought based on what they'd seen so far with the echocardiogram and the EKGs. In fact, I was told my heart itself was healthy and beating normally, though perhaps slightly thick on the left side.

The reason I was getting the *cath procedure* was to get a picture of the "overall landscape" of my heart prior to surgery. This way, they could fix anything else that needed it while I was lying there opened up like a sardine can. But, of course, if anything was discovered that could be remedied as part of an angiogram, they were going to do what they could then and there.

They make a big deal out of preparing for an angiogram. In fact, they sent me this package in the mail that had a brochure and a bunch of information on what this was all about and what to expect. Problem is, the package arrived the day *after* I'd had it done. Ah well, at least they tried. But I was prepared enough by my usual self-education on the matter, as well as a detailed note from my cardiologist.

A quick blurb on these brochures. They really crack me up. Each page has a picture of people, usually a bit older, late 50s through 70s, smiling away at the camera. I mean they're just so happy or even laughing about something. I get the psychology behind it all; I've done marketing and copyrighting. You're not going to show scared people or someone in pain on these things. But still, the grins and laughter? Come on, like we're all so happy that a surgeon is about to cut me open and mess with the most important organ of the body, save the brain. If I were designing these things, I'd have at least one more serious looking photo of someone talking to a doctor, but that's just me.

The research I did prior to this angiogram procedure once again did me more harm than good. But I still had to do it. What I mean by that is, I learned what the approximately 11 things are that can go wrong—the top three being heart attack, stroke, and death—similar risks I was facing with the surgery. Lesser items included arteries tearing from the catheter and allergic reactions to the dye.

But I didn't bother expressing any of these concerns to my doctors or the staff for two reasons. The first was that this had to be done, so whining about what could go wrong would not stop or change anything. Well, I *could* have cancelled everything including the surgery and take a "right to refuse treatment" approach. If I was already 80 years or older, I probably would have, but I wasn't going to do that at this point. Secondly, they'd have given me the same answer they always do, that while those risks are real, they happen only to a "very small percentage" of unlucky folks. They never use words like 'unlucky,' of course, but that's really what it comes down to. My glass-half-empty mentality always says things like, *well, someone has to be in that small percentage, why not me?* But again, thinking like that is futile, and by the way, this whole experience would actually help me get better in some ways with regards to negative thinking. I'll go over that later.

So after checking in at the "pre-op" station at the hospital, my info was taken and I filled out a consent form. After all, what I was doing could result in me never walking out of the place again, not of my own accord anyway. Whatever happens, it said, I know the risks and my family can't sue the hospital.

To be fair, when I went skydiving years before in my Roaring 20's, the papers I had to read and sign were much more ominous—quite intimidating and almost over-whelming, really. Page after page, a small booklet actually, of legal talk that came down to this: *You understand that what you're doing is risky and could result in extreme pain, suf-fering, paralysis, death and everything in between. And if any of that happens, neither you nor your family can hold us respon-sible.* Seriously. Yeah, I did the skydiving anyway, but I was 24 and a different person then. I had a lot less to lose. The consent form I signed at the hospital was only a two-pager, but it basically said the same things.

After a few minutes, a tech came out to the waiting room and called my name, young guy in his early 20's. He took me down the hall and after taking my weight, tem-perature, and blood pressure on both arms, escorted me to a large room where lots of patients were waiting for all types of procedures. The "bed stalls" were just spaces separated by draw curtains and once in my private space, I was told to remove everything, including underwear, and place it in these bags they had ready—one for the shoes and the other for everything else.

The room was cold and the floor was the usual hard tile hospital style, so it wasn't very pleasant. But they did have these anti-slip socks, same kind I wore for the MRI, and they felt kind of good.

Because we were all divided only by thin curtains, I could hear the conversations around me. I wasn't eavesdrop-ping, you could just hear things. Some lady next to me was getting major surgery and the doctor was marking her skin where they were going to do the cutting. Another person next to me was getting their gall bladder removed. None of it mattered to me, I had enough to ponder on myself.

Finally a nurse showed up who put things on me that would remain my whole stay, all on my left arm: an IV in the back of my hand, an oximeter taped to my thumb, and a cuff that would automatically check my blood pressure every couple minutes, when hooked up. She was a docile and quiet woman in maybe her early 40's who, thankfully, didn't try to make a lot of conversation. But what I really remember about her is that after she found out why I was there and what I was preparing for (open-heart surgery), she gave me a sad look and said, "Oh, only 49 and you have to do this?"

"Yep," I said turning away, sullenly. "That's my life right now."

I said this with some bitterness and it made her pause. I wasn't bitter at her and wasn't trying to direct anything at her. It wasn't her fault I was there. I was more bitter at circumstances in general. I know she wasn't trying to be mean or even gush unwanted pity, she was just being honest in her response to my situation.

I suppose a comment like that from anyone, much less a medical professional, would have hit me harder a month or two before this. But I'd done much research and I found stories of lots of people much younger than me that had been through this. Some as young as their early 20's, some children, due to things they were born with. My wife and I also know a single mom whose baby, only three as of this writing, whose has had numerous surgeries due to birth problems. So at this point, although cynical, I wasn't going to leap too far down the hole of self-pity, tempting as it was.

Then I was asked about a ride home. I told her I'd taken a rideshare in and that I was planning to take it back. Oh no, that wasn't a possibility, I was told. Somebody you know must give you a ride. That was their policy.

Now, my wife is absolutely wonderful and supportive and everything I could possibly want or need. She'd offered to take time off work and her busy after-school tutoring to be with me on this day. But I'd insisted she not take me and just stick to her regular schedule. So this was my fault.

I tried to say look, I don't live far away, not even a 15-minute drive. No, I was told. If I didn't have a ride back they were going to cancel the whole thing. Sigh…Okay, so I gave them my wife's name and number and they were going to call her. I would have to just hope she could make it when I was finished. Maybe I could still trick them and say my wife was coming but then just call a ride when I got out front. This, I would find out, wasn't going to work.

After the nurse finished, along came someone with a portable EKG machine. Nice lady who smiled a lot and tried to be as genuinely pleasant as possible as she stuck electrode stickers all over me. I'd just been through this a couple weeks ago so I knew what to expect. Knowing in advance that something is painless or not a big deal always helps.

When that was over and a few more of my chest hairs were ripped out by stickers, a nurse practitioner came by with a portable workstation and asked a whole other set of questions, mainly about my family's medical history. She then went into a detailed description of what a coronary angiogram entailed. Although I'd watched several videos of the whole angiogram experience and knew most of it, I patiently nodded as she went through the procedure. But I did learn a couple new things.

So here's how it works. They cut open an artery in either your wrist or your groin area. They want to try the wrist first because it's less dangerous and heals faster. So the wrist method is, of course, what I was hoping would work me. But they don't know what's going to happen until you're there in the procedure room and making the attempt. Arteries, as I've said, carry blood from your heart and are subject to much higher pressures than veins, so cutting them is always risky.

After successfully getting into your artery, they insert an "introduction" devise which is basically a small, elongated funnel which helps the long, thin, catheter—a rubber or plastic tube—into your body. The doctor pushes the catheter all the way up into your heart and near or into your coronary arteries, depending. Once there, a specialty iodine dye is released into your blood that makes it easier to see the arteries in every detail through the x-ray machine hovering over your chest. From there, they can see if there are any blockages causing blood not to get to certain parts of your heart. If they find nothing wrong, you're a lot safer in terms of risks and complications than if they have to do any intervention.

If they do find any blockages, there's two things they might be able to do to have you avoid surgery, but it depends on if they can get the catheter squeezed into the opening where the obstruction is (I was going to have surgery anyway, but no problems here meant one less thing to fix). The first is that they have a little balloon on the end of the catheter. After wedging the deflated balloon where the impasse is, they gently inflate it so that it stretches the artery walls apart and creates a wider area for blood to flow.

The second thing they may be to do, if the artery is collapsed or hardened and doesn't want to stay open, is put in a stent. Now it's a procedure called *percutaneous coronary intervention*. Why? Because doctors love fancy names for stuff. Another name that's a little easier is *angioplasty*.

A stent is a tiny expandable tube made of woven steel. The balloon on the catheter is inside the collapsed stent which is placed where the blockage is in the artery and then inflated. This causes the stent to expand and then stay in place. The catheter is then removed and the stent stays in you, for life. They coat stents with drugs that help your body not reject them.

Lots of people get stents. As of this writing, presidential candidate Bernie Sanders recently had two stents put in after suffering a heart attack on the campaign trail. A couple years before this, a friend of mine had been going along in what was an otherwise normal day when he suddenly felt chest pains. They weren't that bad, but they were there. He also felt winded and tired. He sat by the bed waiting for the feeling to go away but after three or four hours, the feelings persisted. Finally, at the urging of his wife, they went to emergency. A couple hours later he was rushed somewhere, where they put in two stents. He was told he was having a type of "slow" heart attack that goes for a while before eventually killing you. He came close.

Does one have to take anticoagulant drugs like Warfarin/Coumadin after getting stents? Most take them for at least a year after such implants, yes. But there are different kinds of stents, coated vs. bare metal, that require more or less of this sort of thing. At a minimum, one would have to take some kind of dual anticoagulant and aspirin for while anyway.

Back to me…The nurse practitioner squeezed my wrist tightly in several places and then commented that she saw my skin turn "nice and pink," meaning there was a good chance they'd be able to go through my wrist rather than my groin. The difference is that the artery near the groin (the femoral) is bigger and the blood flow is more powerful. This means there's more chance of bleeding afterwards and it takes longer to heal. And the difference is substantial. If they go in through the wrist and arm arteries (the radial to the brachial), you have to sit in a bed and be monitored for two to three hours, typically. But if they go in through the groin, you have to lie flat on your back and not move for four to six hours and be monitored.

Wrist, God, please. Let them be able to use my wrist.

I was also told I'd be given a sedative to relax me, but would not induce sleep. I'd heard about the sedative from videos I'd seen and descriptions I'd read, but for some reason this didn't comfort me. I didn't want to go home blathering, drugged-up and feeling nauseous from the anesthesia. But again, did I have a choice?

The nurse practitioner wished me the best (no guarantees) and then left. I laid there for another 30 or 40 minutes listening to nurses bustle around and doctors come and go to the patients. These moments are the worst because of the anticipation. You hear doctors around you trying to reassure their patients how they're going to do everything possible, that there's a *very good chance* everything will be fine and so on. But everyone is on edge there, you can feel it in the air, a high-energy tension. At least most, unlike me, were trying to be positive about it. You reach a point though to where you just want them to start cutting and get it over with.

Finally, a technician came along and told me they were ready for me. She was Asian, and one of those individuals that looked 30, but was probably closer to 50. I didn't ask. She said *Hi* and introduced herself, but I was blanking out and don't remember her name. She un-braked my bed and we started down a series of hallways and in an elevator to the floor below. Along the way she was chatting nonchalantly and rather noisily with another nurse or someone about vacation spots and kids applying for college. The college-bound kids talk confirmed my suspicions about my tech's age. They did a lot of laughing. I don't blame them, but once again, I was reminded that I was merely patient number 5,001 and this was all just routine.

Don't get me wrong, no one was treating me like I was *just a number* or that I was imposing on them. They see patients come and go all day, every day. But despite this, most were actually doing their best to be amiable. As with any situation in life, some people are good-natured and some are not.

I'd been a little tainted years ago when my first child was born. There was a nurse there who'd been impatient and snappy with my wife which really unhooked my humor. She was older, greying hair and maybe on the verge of retiring and was done. But I couldn't say anything because it wasn't me who was enduring the suffering of first trying to give birth and then having to go through an emergency C-section afterward. So a part of me perhaps expects hospital staff to be at least a little annoyed at the endless stream of patients coming through.

I bring this up to also make that point that at such moments, you're reminded that any misgivings you have that you're more special than anyone else around you goes right out the window. You're not entitled to better treatment. You're not any different than the sick and suffering person next to you. Everyone there has a story and everyone just wants to get better and go home. We're all in the same boat, and I commend hospital staff who take that extra little effort to smile, say hi, and ask every patient how they're doing. It makes a difference.

I remember details of that little trip down the various hallways for a variety of reasons. Mainly, out of all the tests and whatnot that I'd done so far, this was by far the riskiest. And reality was sinking in fast of what I was gearing up for. The last several weeks had flown by quickly, which meant the next several weeks leading up to the operation were going to fly just as fast. There was no getting around it. It wasn't a dream I was going to wake up from. In fact, it was a dream I might never wake up from. Oh, there I go again...

As we rolled along, I remember looking at myself in the hallway intersection mirrors. Down one long corridor, there were windows along one side. My focus went back and forth from the view outside to my reflection as we rolled along, and seeing myself in the hospital bed was surreal. The people outside on the sidewalks were walking their dogs or going to get lattes and didn't have to think about open-heart surgery. Or who knows, maybe some were. Maybe some were thinking about a loved one getting cancer treatment or something else in the floor above mine. You never know what people are going through. I just had a little moment of envy that they were out there and I was in here.

When the elevator doors opened to where they perform the angiograms, the temp seemed to drop another five degrees, and it had already been chilly. A portly woman with bright, red hair, in probably her mid to late 50's behind a desk very cheerfully said, "Is that Mr. Kelly? 'bout time!"

She walked over to where they'd parked me and very friendly-like introduced herself as Nora. I will never forget the 90 minutes or so I spent with Nora and her team down there in those cold rooms. She tried so hard to be humorous and laidback and set my mind at ease, but not in a phony way. She was genuine, and spoke loudly and clearly. And she could tell I was not happy to be there (or had been told) and was doing her best to lessen the tension I was feeling.

As part of the chit-chat, she told me she'd actually started this "cath lab" over 13 years ago and that I was in the best of hands. Well okay, you'd expect her to say that, right? But again, there was an authenticity about her. She was 100% comfortable in her own skin and doing her noblest to make me a little more comfortable too.

Nora then introduced me to the doctor, a gentleman in his early to mid-50s, last name of Shah. He was pleasant and quiet-mannered, but much more straight to the point than Nora. No small talk. He briefly described the procedure and what to expect, assuring me that they *usually* are able to go through the wrist, and then asked me if I had any questions. At this point I did not. He then disappeared down the hall.

After a few minutes, Nora came by with a shaver. It was a standard handheld electric deal but with a really small head. She told me she was going to shave my wrist where they were going to go in. Oh, and in case they were not able to go in through the wrist, she would have to shave "the other part" as well. She said this with a wicked but playful grin and a wink which actually managed to put a smile on my face.

"There, I got a smile!" she exclaimed.

So after shaving my wrist, she carefully lifted the hospital gown just enough so that I wasn't fully exposed and while working the side nearest to center, said, "Don't worry, that's the closest I'll come to the jewels." She really was quite a character.

After a few more minutes, I was told they were ready. *What kind of music do you like?* I was asked. I said classic rock or classical, whatever is easiest.

Nora went into the room and I heard her tell the team, "We've got classic rock today!" Someone chuckled.

It was time.

My bed was wheeled into a larger and even colder room, it seemed, with bright lights and all manner of high-tech looking contraptions on movable arms and tracks hanging from the ceiling. To the left of the bed was a wall of monitors that would rival a modern police station's security console. The place made the dentist's office look like kid's playhouse.

They positioned my bed up to another padded bed, this one stationary. Nora got a heated blanket and draped it over this bed and then they, a team of four now, had me scoot myself over onto it. It was a little harder than the movable bed but otherwise okay. The main thing about this bed was that I had to lie completely flat, no pillow or raise to it. I was warned it may be uncomfortable because of that. In any case, I wasn't going to complain, I just wanted to get this over with. In the background I could hear The Steve Miller Band singing about *flying like an eagle,* and I wondered if the drugs they were about to give me would make me feel like that.

For whatever reason, it didn't occur to me until then that they'd never asked me if I preferred the right wrist to the left to go in. I probably didn't have a choice, but you know how you go in for a flu shot, they ask if want it in your left or right shoulder? I usually choose the right arm because I am left-handed. So in this in case I was almost grateful they were going into the right arm. After all this was done, I would, in fact, be very grateful for their use of my right wrist because it would take some time to heal, which I'll go into.

I'll throw in a blurb here that two days after this procedure I did some more reading up and it turns out that way back in 1989 when they first started performing this procedure, they did, in fact, go in through the left side. And apparently, the left side has some advantages for various reasons, and it made it easier for doctors to learn the techniques. But over time the right side had become the standard simply because most laboratory setups make it easier for the doctor to stand to the right. As well, most of the equipment has traditionally been on the left, for whatever reason. And that was true in my case. Most of the big machines as well as the display monitors were to my left. Of course, they could have just turned me around on the bed, but what do I know, that may have screwed up the x-ray monitor.

The next few minutes were the most intimidating. It's bad enough lying naked, save for the flimsy gown, on a table in a chilly room full of strangers. But when they start strapping you in, that's when it really gets uncomfortable. To be fair, when it started, someone draped another warmed blanket over me which helped, but I was still getting systematically immobilized.

First a small table was wheeled in next to me and my right arm was placed on it, palm up. Then a thick piece of tape was wrapped around my palm, strapping it securely to the table. My nicely trained upbeat mind immediately thought of lethal injection recipients and how they must feel.

Then a tech, or whoever he was, some tall, slender guy in maybe his late 20s, began smearing a gooey substance on my wrist. "Cold," he said, as warning, right before he did it.

Not that I had any time to react and couldn't have done much anyway, but yes, it was indeed cold. He then said "cold" again and did the same thing to my upper thigh/ groin area which was now shaved smooth by Nora. This was, well, a *cold reminder* that that's where they were going to cut me if the wrist didn't work.

While this was happening, the Asian woman rewrapped the blood pressure cuff on my left bicep nice and snug and then attached a short wire to it from one of the many big machines around me. I noted that this immediately limited my movement, especially when it was squeezing. At this point, I couldn't have reached up to scratch my nose with either hand if I'd wanted to.

Then they lowered a big cloth-covered contraption over my chest, the x-ray. It moved on a robotic arm attached to the ceiling. Its shape sort of resembled a big computer monitor, but the older thick, heavy ones, like the Sun monitors we used in the late 90's and early 2000's. This, I would find out, could move in any direction and at any angle while going back and forth over me in small quarter circles.

To complete the feeling of being in a movie about human medical experiments, they stuck one of those two-pronged oxygen nose things into my nose. Okay, it's called a *nasal cannula*, but 'two-pronged nose oxygen thingy' works too.

With my arms secured and big machinery inches from my chest, I was once again in that helpless state I'd felt in the MRI contraption. If I panicked, I could have kicked a bit, that was it. The difference here was that I could see around me, sort of, and Nora and the others could talk to me. I say sort of because that huge thing above my chest blocked most of my view.

Another thing that blocked my view was a cloth or sheet of some kind propped up by little stands someone placed just to my right so that I couldn't look at my wrist during the procedure. Just as well—who wants to look while they cut into you and shove a small tube up your arm? Out of curiosity, I know I would have looked if that little shield wasn't there.

Then I heard Nora tell the Dr. Shah that it's time to scrub-up. He'd been in an adjacent room that I'd not noticed until that moment. I looked to my right past the sheet and saw him come out while Nora and the other techs got his gown, gloves, mask and other items and begin putting them on him.

Once they began, I noticed that he would say something to someone and then whoever he said it to would repeated it. I deduced this was a safety procedure that ensured the person being spoken to had heard and interpreted the instructions correctly. Case in point, when it came time to give me one of the drugs through the IV, he said something to Nora about 125 ccs of this or that and after a moment, she repeated 150. He then corrected her and said, no, 125. She joked something about, *don't listen to me.*

This went on for a few minutes while I patiently waited for the drugs to kick in. And disappointingly, they never did, or at least it didn't seem like it. I was looking around at what I could, waiting for my vision to change a little or to be feeling something, but honestly, I felt nothing.

When it was time to really start, the doctor asked me the standard "safety" questions, a routine I was starting to get used to. He asked me my name, my birth date, and the reason why I was there lying on the bed in that cold room. I dutifully answered, but in retrospect, I should have said that I was there to get a sex change operation. I know Nora would have gotten a kick out of it. But at the time I was just too anxious to attempt humor.

I still didn't feel the drugs in my brain, but I did feel something on my wrist. The doctor began pushing and prodding and then said, "A little burning and stinging."

Then I felt the needle. It felt like a rather long needle as it dug deep and then deeper into the center of my wrist, an inch or so below the palm. This was the pain killer he was going to inject into my wrist. It reminded me of years ago when I went to the dentist and had my upper right wisdom tooth removed. The dentist had stuck a needle into the roof of my mouth which was most unpleasant. But it's that necessary step to making sure you weren't in agonizing pain for what they were about to do next.

A warm, numb feeling began to overtake most of my forearm. Then the next few moments went by kind of quickly as I closed my eyes and tried to focus on the music. I could feel sensations on my wrist as the doctor was pressing around finding just the right place to cut into the artery. Apparently he found it, because the next thing I heard him say was something about "going in."

Okay, so I passed the first big hurtle of them being able to use my wrist artery, not my groin's. One bullet dodged, several more to go.

Still, I waited for the sedative to make me feel different, but couldn't tell what if any of the effects were. Even at the dentist's when you're given nitrous oxide, aka 'laughing gas,' you can feel its effects. And this point I was looking forward to feeling something. It was almost a letdown. But in retrospect, there's a good chance I may have felt something to some degree as the catheter made its way up my artery toward my heart.

I was told that one of the drugs was some sort of relaxant that didn't allow the artery to collapse upon the catheter. Apparently, one of the many defenses the body has is that if it feels a foreign object where it shouldn't be, like something slithering up an artery for example, it tries to stop it. Well that's good.

This is where things got weird. What you experience here is not what I would call pain, just an odd and uncomfortable sensation that was more like an internal pressure. You know those long, skinny balloons clowns use at kid's parties to twist and tie into various shapes and such? Imagine one of those balloons, or perhaps a bicycle tire, in the middle of your arm getting blown up. That's what it felt like. An inside force from the wrist to almost the shoulder which turned into an uncomfortable ache. Nothing agonizing or unbearable, just an uneasy sensation that after a few minutes you start wishing would end. Starting from the shoulder and on up in my chest though, I felt nothing.

After a few minutes I heard the doctor say something about injecting the dye, though he didn't call it "dye." I just deduced this. I had been warned that when the iodine dye is injected, two sensations can result. One is a surge of warmth in the heart area and the other is the intense urge to urinate. I felt neither.

During all this, the big contraption over me was moving around, back and forth, and at one point positioned itself to the right and I was able to glance up at the screens to my upper left. Indeed, I could see the pulsating, dark, inky colored root looking things that were my coronary arteries. Surreal, but yet real.

A few more minutes of this and it was over. We'd only gone through four or five songs on the classic rock track, I think. I heard the doctor say something about no blockages found, although he put it slightly different terms, and then after a moment, "Okay, I'm out."

The next picture is a still image from my actual angiogram procedure. It's actually very interesting to see the video of it because you can see the veins moving and jerking with the heartbeat.

Video still image: Coronary angiogram

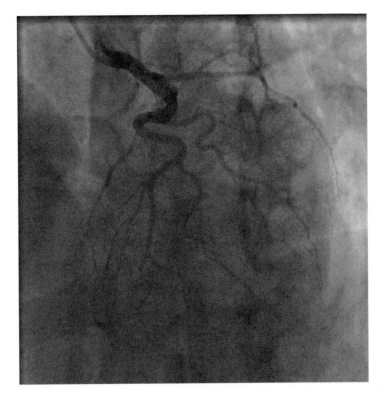

Image source: Kelly Libatique (n.d.). No Copyright.

"I'm out" doesn't sound like something a doctor would say after pulling a catheter out of someone's arm, but it could have been. Maybe it was the drugs I thought I couldn't feel. The point is that several positive things had happened which humbled me and threw cold water, as it were, on my bleak and pessimistic attitude about what was going on that day.

The first was that they had been able to go through the artery in my wrist rather than my groin. This was not only safer, but in practice, meant a quicker recovery. Assuming nothing went wrong, of course. The second was that during the whole procedure, nothing negative happened other than the usual uncomfortable stuff I'd experienced that everyone does. That brochure I'd received a day late that had all the happy, smiley people gave information about strokes and heart attacks, among other things, none of which had happened. The third and one of the biggest was that there were no problems with my coronary arteries that needed fixing. This is huge. Thousands of people need blockages unclogged or bypasses put in which adds to the risks and complications, but I needed none of that. I now knew what others like my friend and even famous folks like David Letterman and Bill Clinton had gone through.

At some point while they were unstrapping me, I asked Nora if they had even given me any drugs. She assured me they had. I looked around and Dr. Shah had disappeared back into his little adjacent room. After a few more minutes, and when it was time for me to get moved back to my portable hospital bed, I got to go for a ride.

"This is the best part," I heard Nora say.

Unbeknownst to me, one of the things they'd put me on was a blow-up blanket of some kind. I heard a hiss of compressed air, like a life raft getting blown up, and suddenly I felt lifted in the air. Not high or anything, just four or five inches maybe. Nora and the team then each grabbed a corner and hoisted/slid me pretty easily back to the portable bed. It was then deflated.

The angiogram was over and now it was time for recovery.

Because of the local anesthetic, I hadn't felt it when the doctor or one of the techs had put this specialty wrist band on me designed specifically for use after this procedure. It was a clear, plastic deal that had a little air hose attached that they use to pump it up tight. And I mean *tight*. I was hardly aware of it until I was wheeled up to a recovery area where I was assigned a nurse who was dedicated just to little'ol me for the next couple hours.

I should mention that Nora herself wheeled me back upstairs to the recovery room. I asked her why and she said she likes to keep an eye on her patients because "shift happens." Makes sense I guess, sticking a tube up someone's artery into their heart, you're seriously messing with nature. When the elevator doors opened, some maintenance or janitorial guy was in there. Without missing a beat, Nora said to him in a brassy and commanding voice, "Patient coming through, out of the way please."

He quickly obliged and stepped out of the elevator. When the elevator doors shut, Nora grinned and said, "You should have seen the look on his face. I've been down here the longest and I'm the meanest nurse here."

The comment kind of surprised me. She'd been anything but mean to me. But then she had that strength and confidence and I could see her not hesitating to blast someone who did something wrong, didn't obey some protocol, or especially put a patient at any unnecessary risk. I think the reason Nora had made such an impression on me is the fact that she truly *owned* her role there at the hospital. It wasn't just a job for her, it was one of her purposes for living.

After Nora dropped me off in the recovery room, she bid me farewell and reminded me not to use my right arm for *anything*. I looked at her face to see if she meant any mischievous double-meaning to that statement, but didn't see any. I gave her a small wave goodbye.

Another nurse, probably mid-30s, was right there and said she'd be keeping an eye on me. She introduced herself as Andrea and began hooking me up to things like the automatic blood pressure machine. But her main focus was the wrist band. She kept checking it every couple of minutes to ensure there was no bleeding.

As Andrea checked, she tried making light conversation. She made the comment that she'd heard I didn't want to be here doing this and was trying to cheer me up. This, I guess, explains why Nora had been trying so hard to put smile on my face. I'm guessing the nurse practitioner who saw me earlier during the prep had told everyone that *we have an unhappy one*, or something to that effect.

Now that I've admitted as much, I need to defend myself a little. I was not in any way, shape, or form trying to give any of the staff an attitude or be unpleasant to them. I felt no negative feelings toward any of them personally. I've seen patients in hospitals be rude and demanding to nurses or other staff and I don't like that. These folks are just doing their jobs. I wasn't being bad-mannered to anyone, scout's honor. I was even making it a point to say *thank you* whenever anyone gave me anything or did something for me.

But I *was* clearly despondent. I confess, I was reeling in self-pity, not so much because of this particular procedure I was doing, but for the overall picture. My negative energy was being focused on myself. I was here as part of the preparation for the most invasive and dodgy of open-heart surgery and it was really weighing heavily on me.

Andrea was trying to be sympathetic and encouraging and all, I'll give her that. At one point she made some comment that made me smile and she said something similar to what Nora had a few minutes earlier, "There's a real smile!"

Clearly, when you work for a hospital, there's training involved in trying to comfort people. After all, people are there because something's wrong. They'd rather be at home, but their bodies are betraying them or some disease is attacking them or they're victims of an accident. They're now confined to a bed, in pain or general discomfort or full of invasive drugs. And often, as is human nature, we take out lousy feelings on the very people around us who are trying to help. Knowing this, I was doing my best not to make anyone's job more difficult than it already must be. In fact, I had been told by someone, Nora, I think, that I had a calm, easy way of talking and she'd asked me if I was a lawyer or some other similar professional. This cracked me up.

Anyway, as time went on, something odd was happening to my right hand. I noticed that the round, fleshy part of the palm where the thumb joint is, started going numb. Then the numbness climbed to the center of my palm and worked its way up the back of my middle finger. A very odd feeling. This alarmed me a little and I told Andrea about it. She and another male nurse started looking at it and were concerned blood flow was getting lost due to the tight wristband thingy. So they put an oximeter on my thumb and verified there was indeed oxygen saturation. They concluded it was a nerve getting pinched by the wristband and it would clear up when it was taken off.

By now the band was starting to hurt, in part because I was focusing more on it at this point. To boot, the local anesthesia was starting to wear off. I can't even imagine a larger version of this tight air-filled band on my thigh if they had had to go through my groin artery. Well, I actually can imagine it now, and the thought was pretty awful.

The good news is that I wasn't bleeding at all. "Not a drop," Andrea said a couple times.

They called Dr. Shah and gave him my status and he said to take the band off in 30 minutes if there was still no bleeding. This was terrific news. Many people have to sit there for two to three hours until the band gets taken off; I'd only been there maybe 20 minutes so far.

Andrea told me that they take post angiogram monitoring very seriously because of the many things they've seen happen to patients afterwards. Severed arteries are dangerous; your own heart can kill you pretty quickly by pumping all your blood out.

My glum thoughts were distracted when Andrea asked if I wanted something to eat. I had completely forgotten that I was told they were going to offer me food. Makes sense since they ask you not to eat starting from the night before. It suddenly occurred to me that I was, in fact, a little hungry.

"Sure," I said. "What do you have?"

She listed out some breakfast items but since it was close to noon the lunch stuff would probably be ready. I didn't feel like anything sweet and sticky so I asked for a sandwich and even got my choice of drink. I chose a cran-apple juice kind of thing. The other nurse kept an eye on me while she went off to get my meal. When she returned, she placed a tray on my lap and put a napkin under my chin.

"Nice being waited on, right?" she asked. I had to agree.

The meal wasn't bad actually—a chicken salad sandwich, a little quinoa salad, and an even smaller "salad" which I put in quotes because it was literally a little tear of lettuce with two slices of cucumber and one cherry tomato. But all this with a yogurt, a small blueberry muffin and the drink and I was more than happy. I didn't realize how hungry I was until I started eating and I was very glad the sedative I was allegedly given wasn't making me sick to my stomach.

Another thing that was really going for me is the fact that again, I'm left-handed. This is good because I was under strict orders to not move my right arm or especially wrist, the one that had been assaulted with the catheter. I can just imagine all the normally right-handed people trying to eat with their left arm both pierced with the IV and wrapped tight by the blood pressure cuff. It was challenging for me and I'm used to my left hand, obviously.

While eating, Andrea took a little device like a large plastic syringe and hooked it to the air hose on the wristband and let out a certain amount of air. This eased the tension a little, but the numbness remained which was starting to bother me. I didn't complain though—just a few more minutes; I was keeping an eye on the wall clock.

After another five or ten minutes, she let out a little more air and this time I could really feel the squeeze easing off. I started to feel a little of the numbness disappearing which was nice, but at the same time, the anesthesia was wearing off and I was feeling an aching pain. The really good news was that there was still no blood. If there had been, that wristband wasn't going to go anywhere.

We chatted a bit during this time, or at least she attempted coaxing me into conversation, trying to comfort me in my decision to have surgery. She said something I won't forget: *I'm proud of you for taking the initiative to take care of yourself.* My wife had also said that, and it made me give myself a little pat on the back.

It makes sense that one of the frustrating things about being in the medical field is seeing patient after patient whose there because they waited too long. They didn't take a doctor's or nurse's advice a long time ago to change or fix something, and now a much worse event or series of events had happened. I liken it to a car. If your mechanic tells you that this or that is about to break down, do you take that long road trip to the middle of nowhere without fixing things? Some people do take chances like that, but I wasn't going to with my aorta and valve in as bad a shape as they were in.

At five minutes till time to remove the wristband, Andrea withdrew even more air from the wristband and relief finally started to come. Slowly but surely, I could start to feel my hand again. I've heard stories of people who get injuries to their hands where nerves are permanently severed and parts of their hands or certain fingers go numb. I now know what that feels like and I wouldn't want the feeling to be permanent. You could be trying to hold something, or worse, getting cut or burned and not feel it.

Well, the top of the hour finally came and Andrea put an absorbing cloth under my wrist, telling me that during this part some people freak out a little because blood gets all over their blanket. She readied a wad of gauge to stop any bleeding and then took the band off. And guess what? No blood, *not a drop*. Nice. In recent years I had been pretty religious about taking my vitamin D and K, among others, and I attribute my healthy arteries and veins and blood clotting abilities in part to that. Well, except for my aorta, but at this point I'll chalk that up as a birth defect.

Andrea raised my arm above my head and pressed the wad of gauze against the artery incision for a minute or two. Then after giving it one last look, put a large plastic see-through tape of some kind over the gauze to keep it in place. Then she took the regular gauze, the wide, tan-brown colored stuff and wrapped my forearm tightly with it, like a cast. That wasn't too comfortable.

After the dressing was on, she put this contraption on my wrist that was really just a piece of foam-padded plastic that had been curved in a way to hold my wrist in place straight, slightly bent upward when Velcro-ed onto my forearm and palm. It was more like a reminder not to move my wrist around.

Then she called the nurse practitioner over, the same one who'd seen me earlier. This nurse carefully pressed above the incision to check my pulse and asked me a bunch of questions about how I was feeling. The numbness was 90% gone at this point confirming that it'd been a pinched nerve that had caused it rather than a more serious lack of blood flow to the hand.

I was then given strict instructions. No moving my right hand, especially in the motion of bending my wrist in a palm forward motion. That motion, I was told, can re-open the artery. Keep the wrist brace and dressing on until the next day when it was time to shower. Next, no driving for three days. What? Yes, because the action of grabbing the steering wheel and gearshift and whatnot can again, cause bad things to happen. I'd disobey this order the very next day, by the way. *Shhhh.*

Next, will your wife be picking you up? Yes, I assured them. So they'd actually put it in my notes to make sure my wife was on the way. Maybe I could still cheat the system…

Now that the air-filled wristband was off and both the doctor and nurse practitioner had given me the green light, it was time to say goodbye to Andrea and get taken to yet another waiting area, this one for the final preparation to get discharged. Maybe this was called the discharge room, I don't know. Actually, that doesn't sound very pleasant, does it.

This room was similar to the one I'd first been put in—large with multiple bed stalls separated by draw curtains. The atmosphere here was brighter though, less stressful, less tension in the air. Here, people were just waiting to go home after surviving whatever procedure they'd been through.

A cheery nurse with a thick Nigerian accent came by and introduced herself and said she'd be taking care of me. She also said she would be calling my wife to tell her when to come get me. They really were not going to let me take a rideshare back. I could only hope my wife could get me in a timely manner, because I was seriously ready to leave at this point.

I was asked if I wanted a flu shot before I left and I thought, why not? I'd already been stuck and cut all morning, what's one more needle going to do? So the nurse ordered one from the pharmacy. After that she said she'd gotten my wife's voice mail and would have to keep trying. Oh boy.

I'll throw in a little blurb here I'm adding to this section a little while after I originally wrote it. The whole coronavirus thing would hit the state of California just four months or so after this and I was so grateful I had that flu shot. Not because it would have stopped COVID, but because it would help to keep me from not having the regular flu if and when I would get exposed. I was really grateful I said yes to that shot.

After offering the flu shot, the nurse also asked me if I wanted lunch and if so, she'd be happy to go get it. For the first time since I got there, I saw a gap in their communication. At least it was with something that was fairly inconsequential. I could always ask for food anytime, after all. But surprisingly, I said no, thank you. A few short years ago I'd have taken the second meal just because I could. But now I honestly didn't have the appetite and didn't want to waste food. Amazing what aging and heart conditions can do to a person.

I had to wait another almost 30 minutes while my nurse took care of other patients around me. Sometime during all that, they had managed to speak to my wife who was making arrangements to leave work early.

At last, the nurse finally came by to remove the IV, thumb oximeter and un-Velcro the blood pressure cuff. It felt good. She then stuck me with the flu shot needle. After this I was told to walk around the room a couple times to get circulation going. I gladly did so and it felt nice to be out of bed. After that, I could finally put my clothes on again.

"I'm going to call your wife again now," the nurse told me. "I will tell her to meet you outside the emergency entrance in 15 minutes."

I looked at the clock and it was a quarter till noon. The nurse got hold of my wife who said she was on her way. I got lucky. The nurse told her to call back at this number when she was five minutes away. Dang, they really enforced the no self-driving policy. What do single or friendless people do in these circumstances? I guess I could have tried to sneak out the door if they couldn't get hold of my wife, but I'm not a rule breaker like that. Besides, I'm sure that would have put a flag on my patient record and I'd end up hearing about it.

I changed back into my clothes and was feeling so good about the results of the procedure, and the fact that I was getting picked up, I started cleaning out my little stall. I took my gown and walked it to the middle where they had a soiled linens basket.

The nurse saw me and said with a big smile, "Oh, you're cleaning up for us. How nice."

At last the moment came when my wife called and said she was almost there. The nurse then called for a "volunteer" to come get me with a wheelchair. These volunteers had been in and out the whole time taking various people away as they were finished. And I was next!

This lady came along with a wheelchair and I hopped in and was ready to leave. The nurse bid me well and we were finally on our way.

When we got outside, the volunteer asked me to point out the car. I wondered what she would have done if I'd just stood up and walked away saying, *I'm fine, thanks*. Would she have called security? Well, I wouldn't have done that, but I was curious. About that moment though, there was my wife circling around the parking lot. It was a most welcome sight. I pointed out the car and waved and she drove up. What a relief to get up out of that chair, dressed in my own clothes, and get into my own car. These events make you appreciate the little things.

Now on to recovery at home from a coronary angiogram.

I'm not going to lie, my wrist and much of my arm hurt for almost a month afterward. First off, I can understand why they say don't drive for three days. There's an odd feeling of internal damage that happens to one's wrist from this. In fact, even a full two weeks after the procedure, I could feel it, especially if I pressed anywhere within about a six or seven inch distance down my arm from where the doctor went into my artery.

Over the next couple days, the bruising progressively got worse and looked especially ugly on the third day. The part that bruises the most is where you get stuck with the local anesthetic needle though, not where the catheter went in. On day two and three, the bruising is an angry red mixed with the usual black and blue. From there the red slowly dissipates, but the bruising seems to get even bigger for another day or two, working its way down your forearm. Some of it even appeared and made its way around to the back of my hand near my thumb and wrist area. And it was sore to the touch, not terribly so, but you don't want to press on it or worse, accidentally bump it on something.

I was warned not to bend my wrist at all, so I did my best to keep that brace thingy strapped to my hand the first day, but I did have to remove the gauze as it was just too tight and my hand was cold from the circulation getting cut off. They had said don't take it off until tomorrow's shower, but I couldn't take the idea of leaving it on all night. So I pealed it off. No blood seeping through the small taped wad on the wound!

I was told that if it started bleeding, to elevate my wrist, press firmly with two fingers against it and hold for 15 minutes. If the bleeding still wouldn't stop, go to emergency. The thought killed me—another several hours in a hospital. But cutting arteries is serious business.

The following picture is my actual forearm eight days after the angiogram. I should have taken it earlier to show how red it was the first two or three days. Notice the bruising that had formed down my arm.

Number 1 is where they cut into my artery and number 2 is about where the local anesthetic was administered.

Photo: Forearm eight days after the angiogram

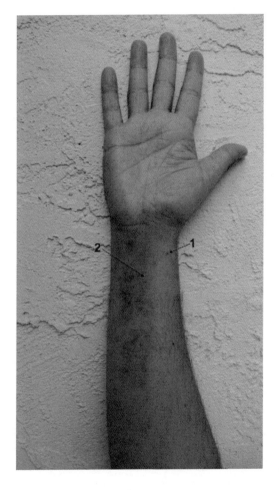

Image source: Kelly Libatique (n.d.). No copyright.

My wrist and arm were very sore until about the start of the second week, especially directly beneath the incision spot (number 1) for several inches. Again, it was an internal damage kind of feeling, a soreness and injury within, not pleasant at all. As for the center of my wrist where the anesthetic was injected, it didn't really hurt if I didn't move it, but if I bent my wrist in either direction, particularly if I bent it backward to stretch my palm outward, it ached very painfully for several minutes. It was like a nerve had been damaged.

It was suggested to take acetaminophen for pain management, which I did a couple times, usually in the morning. Aspirin and ibuprofen are anti-coagulants and you don't want that big bruise to get any larger. One more reason why I was grateful to not be on any drugs like Coumadin.

Also, if I slept in such a way so that weight was put on my arm, it was really sore the next morning. At night I'd wake up having rolled on my right arm without knowing it and when I moved and circulation flowed once again through that arm, the wrist area really ached. At one point I was getting nervous that I'd been infected, but there was no swelling or redness, and I had no fever, so I let it go.

By the end of the second week, the bruising was finally waning. The area that had bothered me the most, the first few inches up my arm from where the catheter was inserted, was finally not as sore to the touch. But the wrist area where the anesthetic had been injected still hurt. Fortunately, the pain was there only when bending my wrist in certain ways or pressing the area.

I watched carefully for signs of infection but still none came. A day or two before this, I had sent a note to my cardiologist asking about valves and he had scheduled a phone conversation. During the talk, I described my forearm and he suggested sending him a picture of it over the secure website. So I did and a day later he said as long as you don't feel any numbness or increasing pain, I should be okay.

Finally, about three weeks after the event, the pain and bruising were about gone, except for if I slept wrong on the arm or bent my wrist at a hard angle. By the end of the fourth week, one wouldn't really notice anything unless it was pointed out. Good timing too because the surgery would only be a week away.

So there you have it. My experience with a coronary angiogram or "cath procedure" really wasn't that bad, just inconvenient. No heart attack, no stroke, and I'm still alive. As with so many of these things, the anticipation is the worst of it. The post procedure recovery was quite bothersome, but I'll take some bruising and pain over a stroke any day.

The Dentist

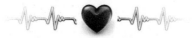

"Teeth are always in style."

—Dr. Seuss

S o at the fine middle-age of 49, I got my first major dental work done. Actually, not true. I did have two wisdom teeth removed about 20 years prior to this and that had been quite an ordeal. A bigger deal actually than what I was about to do. In fact, the general dentist who'd done the work said my bones were so strong, he didn't want to do the two remaining wisdom teeth (it had taken awhile and I'd inhaled a lot of nitrous oxide that morning). If I'd wanted it done, he would refer me to an oral surgeon. Out of both laziness and apprehension, I never had them removed. Now I was paying the price.

I mentioned that in my conversation with Dr. Dan, my surgeon, he told me I needed to see the dentist. My cardiologist had repeated this at some point, but I forget when on the timeline. So I booked a session with the dentist and told them I just needed a cleaning and exam. This was actually a couple weeks before the coronary angiogram.

When I first came in, I didn't say what I was there for. The cleaning went fine and was the usual experience. The dental hygienist did the scouring and buffing as normal.

I hate the part where they scrape up against the gums at the top with that sharp little tool—it always hurts and bleeds a little.

When it was over, the main dentist came in for the final check. We started chatting and he asked why it had been so long since I came in. So I started telling him all about my upcoming adventure on the operating table and that I was told if there was any infections or problems, I needed it taken care of. Additionally, if there was any work that needed doing, he was supposed to give me antibiotics. His eyes got wide and I could tell he got a little alarmed. I explained that the reason I'd not mentioned it until now that I didn't consider a regular cleaning "dental work." I figured that was for a tooth getting pulled or something. Well, he said, there was some bleeding involved just now during the cleaning so we should have done this. He quickly had his assistant grab some amoxicillin and asked if I was allergic to antibiotics. I said no, but years ago when I was a kid, some erythromycin had given me a bad stomachache. So he gave me a double dose of the amoxicillin and said he was going to call my cardiologist.

I felt a little bad—it hadn't been my intention to frighten the dentist.

Now came the surprise. He asked if I had remembered that a couple cavities were just starting to form on my two remaining wisdom teeth. When he mentioned it, I did vaguely remember something about that the last time I was in. But I'd never had cavities in my life and it was one of those things you're told: *This is no big deal now and it can be taken care of in the next several years, or maybe not at all.* Just like Dr. Dan had said dentists were notorious for.

But the cavities, while not yet an issue, had gotten a little deeper since I'd been in two or three years ago. Eventually, they may be problematic. If I wanted to do something now, I had a choice to either have them filled or be referred to an oral surgeon to have the actual teeth removed. I sighed and said, okay, let's fill them in, and we need to get this taken care of ASAP. When was the next appointment? I booked it for about a week and half later.

Filling cavities has changed. There's so many materials now besides the traditional gold and silver. Mine was going to be this composite made from a mix of powered glass and acrylic resin. The advantages is that this stuff bonds with the tooth and can be instantly cured with a special tool. But I wasn't concerned about that. My concern was pain. Would there be drilling and so forth. There was, as it turned out, but not much and nothing that would hit any raw nerves.

The whole filling procedure took about 25 minutes. Other than choking and gagging a couple times on the devices to keep my mouth open and my tongue out of the way, it went pretty smooth. The worst thing that happened was when the drill rubbed against my tongue at some point and caused a little friction burn. This would later turn into a canker sore that lasted about a week. Ah well, just one more inconvenience to deal with as part of the whole process of replacing my aortic root and possibly my aortic valve.

On my way out, the dentist told me a story of how his father in law had had a similar procedure (open-heart surgery) several years ago in Santa Clara and that everything turned out just fine. I thanked him and was grateful for his effort to be encouraging.

The takeaway here is that there's a price to pay for every decision we make. This was especially true in my choice to turn a blind eye to blood pressure and sleep apnea issues. In this case, my two remaining wisdom teeth have caused more problems than they've done me good. Over the years, I've gotten small infections from food getting stuck way back there between the gums and the tooth. Nothing big, a little soreness and swollen gums, but still an inconvenience.

And now these cavities. I could have had these teeth removed years ago and then I wouldn't have had to get them quickly filled in right before surgery. Buried under the layers of our procrastination, there always lurks things that will not go away on their own and in most cases, become worse with time.

Life is so full of these *coulda, shoulda, woulda* scenarios…

The "Pre-op"

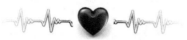

**"Be nice to nurses. We keep doctors
from accidentally killing you."**

—Unknown

My "pre-op" or pre-surgery appointment was scheduled exactly 15 days before the surgery day. Out of all the stuff I had to do to prepare for the surgeon's sawblade, this was the easiest. It was just time consuming and yet another couple hours spent in a hospital.

I'll throw in a quick blurb here to say that one day before this pre-op, I decided to tell my surgeon that if there was no possible way to save my native aortic valve, I had opted for a tissue/bioprosthetic valve over the mechanical. I didn't give any big explanations. I merely said that I'd given it full consideration, understood the short and long term implications, and that it was my wish to avoid a Coumadin-for-life prescription.

I then waited with a bit of apprehension for a response. After all, he was the guy in charge of making major changes in my life and I was going against his recommendations. He had years of experience, and I do believe he was basing his advice on what he thought was best for me, especially with regards to long-term outcomes.

The response came in just a couple hours. My healthcare provider has a great system where via a website, you can send secure email directly to your various doctors. Maybe that's normal anymore for most providers. I'd already used it several times with my regular doctor and cardiologist and found them to be very responsive. It's an effective approach and a far cry from the olden days where you'd call the "department" or main office and leave messages with some call center person and hope it got through all the layers to your doctor in a reasonable amount of time. Then you had to wait for the response to bubble back up through all those layers.

Anyway, my surgeon simply replied that he would do "everything they could" to save my native valve, but if it was not possible, they'd put in a bioprosthetic. He added that he "respected" my decision. No lectures, no, *Are you sure?* I was thankful for that. Now I had to hope I was making the right decision. I did take note that telling someone they respect one's choice is a diplomatic way of saying, *I disagree with you, but will still support you…*

For this pre-op, I had to show up in San Francisco for a 9:00 AM check-in, dead smack dab in the mess of rush hour traffic. Yes, I was griping a little, but more as a cover-up for the fear I was feeling. My wife accompanied me this time and I was grateful for the support.

At this point it had been roughly two months since I'd heard that open-heart surgery was an inevitable reality I was facing. I'd read stories of others who'd been told that similar surgery was going to happen, but much further down the road, months or even years away. In retrospect, I would not want to wait that long—too much anticipation! My situation had been moving along fairly quickly, once the diagnosis had been made in early September. From one test and appointment to the next, this train was moving fast.

The mind has strange ways of distracting itself to reduce stress. Especially in these last couple weeks, I would find my thoughts wandering or I'd spontaneously throw myself into a task and go at it hard so I couldn't think about anything else. Or, I'd think of something funny and milk the laughter and amusing feelings as long as I possibly could before returning to "reality." If I was watching a movie, even if it was just an okay flick, I'd get totally engrossed in the story, more so than I used to. When the movie ended, I would again be thrust back into the thoughts of my situation and all the feelings that came with it.

Anyway, a pre-op is a final check of everything on or in your body before they put you on the cutting slab. I was told there was no sedation for anything so I could drive myself. As well, there was no need to fast for the blood tests so go ahead and have breakfast that morning. I ate a nice, big, *distracting* breakfast.

I had three main appointments that morning, the third of which was meeting and talking to a couple individuals. I'd been told I would have to give a urine sample as part of the lab work, so I deliberately drank a whole coffee-mocha drink on the drive in because I'd been warned this pre-op could take three to four hours; the last thing I wanted to do was sit around and be delayed. The coffee drink worked.

My first appointment was the lab and it was on the second floor. For whatever reason, an eerie feeing came over me as my wife and I took the elevator. I don't know why. I'd been in a similar situation before so many times in the last few weeks. I guess because this was the final preparation, the one where I'd be given instructions on what to do and what to expect on the day of surgery. Up until now, the actual day had been shrouded in mystery. Details like where exactly I go and when and all that had not been given to me yet. They would be soon.

At the lab registration desk, I was met by yet another hurried individual and even though it was still pretty early, I was clearly just the next one in line.

The girl behind the counter, early or mid-20's at the most, punched up my info in the screen and asked with a slight Tagalog accent, "You're having surgery on November 4?" The question could have been an indifferent, "Did you want room for cream and sugar?" I just nodded.

I was handed a form to sign and a bag with a urine sample cup. The restrooms were down the hall, it was pointed out, and then I was told to sit and wait for my number to be called.

After maybe ten minutes my number was called, and when I went back to have my blood drawn, I was surprised at how much they took—five or six of those little vials. I was half expecting to feel dizzy or something but did not. I then went to the restroom, did what I was asked and dropped the bag off at the counter on my way out.

Well, that went pretty fast and easy. Next stop, the x-ray.

X-rays were on the third floor. I looked for stairs and didn't see any so we took another elevator ride. I was feeling a little better already because of how quickly the lab thing went. Maybe I could get out of here early. For this x-ray, I was anticipating having to take off my shirt and lay on a bed or whatever, but that's not what happened.

I registered with the desk and then was called back in about 15 minutes. In a hallway near the x-ray equipment room there were four or five others waiting. A lady in front of me was having an x-ray done on her knee and I'd heard someone tell her to go into a changing room and put on hospital pants. Great, I thought, I'm going to have to change again.

But no, I was directed by another hurried tech into the x-ray room who simply told me to remove my jacket. I'd worn a t-shirt that day and he looked at it for a second and decided that was fine. I was asked to stand in front of this machine that had several panels of different shapes—some flat and rectangular, some curved like arches. All I had to do was stand and face the various pieces of the machine and hold my breath. It took about five seconds. Then I was asked to turn to my right and raise my arms above my head and hold my breath again.

And then it was over. In not even 40 minutes since I'd walked into the place, I was already done with two of three appointments. My naturally cynical mind was beginning to get suspicious that something was missing or a surprise was going to get thrown at me.

Now the final elevator ride to the eighth floor. I knew I was going to meet my anesthesiologist, and this would be a very important person during surgery, in many ways, just as important as the surgeon himself. I registered at the desk and then waited maybe 20 minutes.

I was called back into the hallways by a nurse or technician, but before we went into a room, I was asked to walk a certain distance a couple times. The girl doing it walked away about 30 feet, then had me walk to her as I'd "normally" walk. We did this a couple times back and forth while she watched me, then jotted some notes on a clipboard. She offered no explanation of what this was about. I could have asked, but for some reason, I just wasn't curious enough.

I was then taken into a typical looking doctor's patient room with the exam bed, chairs, workstation and so on. On the wall was a wonderfully illustrated poster that explained the functions of the heart, complete with arrows and descriptions depicting the circulatory flow of blood through a human's body. I would end up occupying my time between interviews by studying this poster.

The same girl who'd had me walk in the hall took my blood pressure on both arms and then my temperature. She then did a quick EKG that involved the electrode stickers on my arms and chest only, no legs this time. I was grateful I didn't have to remove my pants. During all this, I was asked the standard procedure stuff with the usual, *How are you feeling right now?* kind of questions. I was then told to wait for the anesthesiologist. It took ten or 15 minutes for him to arrive and I studied the heart poster during this time.

The next image is a picture of a typical model of a human heart I've seen at my cardiologist's office and other places I've visited. You can take it apart and look at the insides of this amazing organ.

Photo: Model of a heart

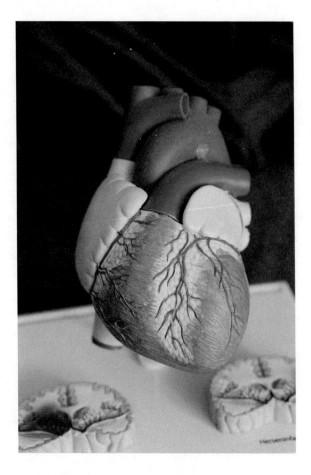

Photo by Robina Weermeijer on Unsplash (May 23, 2020).
Retrieved from https://unsplash.com/photos/NIuGLCC7q54

The anesthesiologist was a young guy in his early 30's and who was the most hurried person I'd run into yet. He clearly had other things to do, but it was his duty to be my upcoming surgery anesthesiology consultation. Despite this, he did give me his attention for the maybe 20 minutes I had him. I also noticed he appeared almost slightly nervous. Maybe it was because I was being very serious—no smiling, no humor; perhaps he wasn't sure how to handle me in that respect. I don't know. For his part, he didn't have an easy going, witty and engaging personality like Nora or some of the other folks had that I'd met along this journey.

He introduced himself as Dr. something or another, but I forgot the name. I think it slipped my mind because one of the first things he told me was that he may not be the actual anesthesiologist who takes care of me the morning of my surgery. I found this to be disappointing, but didn't bother saying that. I wondered if this was standard procedure. I'd been hoping to meet the actual person who was going to put me under and be there at the time because there were certain questions I had and I wanted to feel like I knew the person a little. Now I felt like those questions didn't matter as much. But I got the clarification. He explained that there were four or five anesthesiologists on a rotation for that week and it's easier to get the assignment the morning of rather than book things more than two weeks out. Made sense, I guess.

"Have you ever been under general anesthesia?" he asked. I had not. I would find out later that this is an important question because they want to know if anesthesia had caused any complications before or had made you sick. So in my case, we were just going to have to find out.

He then went on to explain that he personally had experienced general anesthesia for something or another awhile back, and I did appreciate that. I'd rather someone tell me about something from actual experience rather than just theory or a textbook.

He explained that "going under" was essentially a drug induced coma and that I won't remember anything or have any concept of time. I'd heard this before from other's stories. Some say it's like you close your eyes and after what feels like a minute or two, you're coming back around and the surgery is all over. You can't tell if five minutes or five hours had passed.

He went into to some of the descriptions of the various drugs used and the stages, but my mind was now wandering and I didn't hear much. I guess this was in part because I'd already seen videos where the whole anesthesiology process was explained. It was obvious I was reaching a point to where I was tired of gathering intel about all this.

He then mentioned something that snapped me back to the moment. He said that if a blood transfusion became necessary during the surgery, there was a small chance I'd be exposed to hepatitis C or HIV. *Great.* He said it in a way that was clearly legal talk and something they had to do to both warn me and cover themselves. I knew I'd be signing consent forms on the morning of the surgery and one of things I'd be autographing was that I'd been told about this, but was agreeing to the risk anyway. So if anything happened…

I later read somewhere that the risk of exposure to hepatitis or HIV during blood transfusions was low, like 1.8%, and I think Dr. So and So had said as much. In raking my memory, Dr. Dan, my surgeon, may have mentioned this too. But for some reason, that little *Fun Fact* had slipped my mind that morning and I wasn't even thinking about it until I got reminded.

Dr. So and So looked at me for an extra moment to gauge my reaction and all I did was stare at him with what was probably an expression of both fear and alarm. So he followed up by saying that he's worked with my particular surgeon many times and there had never been a need for a transfusion, at least with Dr. Dan. One would think everyone who gives blood is screened for all of this, but I guess not. Either that or some just slip through the cracks. Scary, but true.

The rest of our interview was mainly about preexisting health conditions, the same questions I'd been answering for weeks. Fortunately, most of my answers were in my favor—that I'd never had cancer or diabetes or a number of other things which can complicate general anesthesia or surgery. So I didn't mind answering them again.

Grabbing a pen light, he then asked me to open my mouth wide so he could have a look. I obliged and he explained that there's a device they use to put the breathing tube down my throat and he wanted to make sure the back of my mouth looked normal. He assured me that I'd be out during this and not feel it. I didn't say it, but thought, *you'd better be right about that.* I've seen videos of people getting intubated while still conscious and the thrashing and choking they do looks horrifying.

He then mentioned something else which made me uneasy. In an all nice and lawyer-like way again, he said that during intubation, when the breathing tube is inserted, there's a small chance of tracheal or esophageal perforation. Apparently, in certain cases, the tube can inadvertently pierce or puncture your throat during placement. This, of course, can not only asphyxiate you, but can result in life-threatening internal bleeding. He quickly added that it's rare though and usually the result of a patient having other preexisting conditions. This story just kept getting better and better.

After that he finished with, "Well, that's all I've got, any questions?" I said no.

Now he wanted to take a quick listen to my heart and lungs. He listened carefully with a stethoscope while I took big breaths in and out and then made some notes in the workstation. I asked him if he'd heard the heart murmur just now and he said he had not. He said that whoever had, had "good skills" in that area (kudos for my general/internal medicine doctor). But then, apparently misunderstanding me, he quickly followed-up by saying that due to the aneurism, I should still proceed with the surgery. I told him I wasn't trying to weasel out of anything at this point; I'd succumbed to fate. I was just curious. He quickly smiled as best as he could, told me a nurse practitioner was on her way, and then hurried out the door, the long end of his white coat swirling like a cape. *See ya, doc.*

One of the questions I had wanted to ask about but did not was the phenomena of what's called *anesthesia awareness*. It's sometimes also referred to as 'intraoperative awareness' or 'accidental awareness.' That's when you "wake up" and become conscience while they're cutting into you, hammering a rod in your leg, or whatever. Apparently, less than 1% of surgery patients experience this, but that's still thousands of people when you add it up over the years.

This one lady in 1998 in Virginia was having surgery to remove an eye and says she was as alert as any normal time of the day and could feel what has happening to her. She could hear disco music, could sense the pressure and sensations of the tools, and someone telling someone else to "Cut deeper, pull harder." She wanted to scream, cry out, anything, but was totally paralyzed and helpless. When that happens, they call it *explicit recall* because a patient can remember, well, explicit details. It was so traumatic that she lived with PTSD for years. It's the stuff of nightmares.

Fortunately, the drug that kills pain is separate from the drug that puts you under (and separate from the drugs that paralyze you). This is important because if you were both conscience *and* could feel pain, that would be a double failure on the part of the anesthesiologist (or the equipment). But this ghastly scenario *has* happened to an unlucky few and just the thought is enough to make one shudder. Everyone on a surgical team is supposed to be well trained to watch for signs that a patient is coming to, but things obviously happen and go unnoticed by the busy and often stressed people that perform these procedures.

What causes anesthesia awareness can be equipment failure. I've read that full equipment checks are supposed to be done before every surgery, like the way pilots do pre-flight checks. But you know how things go. Humans make mistakes, things get overlooked, people get into a hurry and routine fatigue comes into play. Machines also break down like any other mechanical devices.

But anesthesia awareness can also happen because of something as simple as your anesthesiologist not giving you enough drugs. Sometimes they don't want to give you too much or you'll be sick afterwards, which is especially the case if you've had that happen before. But not just that, certain surgical procedures are apparently more prone to having this happen than others. For example, they don't want to give too much to women undergoing C-sections because they don't want the baby overexposed. My wife was actually almost fully awake during her C-section which was deliberate because it had been an emergency procedure and our son's heart had slowed due to lack of oxygen. She'd felt no pain though, thank God.

Another kind of surgery prone to anesthesia awareness is…can you guess? Yep, heart surgery. It has something to do with keeping the patient stable.

I didn't bother bringing all this up with Dr. So and So because it just didn't feel right. He was in a hurry and all he'd do is give me the standard assurance, in his uneasy and most diplomatic way, that this would not happen to me under his care or at this hospital. I mean really, what else would he possibly tell me? And even if he did admit it had happened here, what would I do, cancel everything? I resolved to bring the subject up on the morning of my surgery though.

In the room alone again, I studied the heart poster. I looked carefully at the aortic valve from the different angles presented and wished so much that life hadn't dealt me this card. But what did wishing ever do for anyone? The heart is an amazing organ, only the size of one's fist and yet it does so much all day, every day to keep a person alive.

A few minutes later there was a knock on the door and a woman, a nurse practitioner, late 30's or early 40's, with a warm smile came in and introduced herself as Joanne. Her job was to explain what I would be expecting and what I was supposed to do, specifically starting about a week before the surgery.

She must have seen the apprehension in my eyes because she pressed with the *how are you doing?* and *how are you feeling?* questions. I finally admitted I was taking this whole thing pretty hard, especially since everything was a first for me. I'd never had any surgery before, except for a couple wisdom teeth, and I'd never experienced general anesthesia. She did and said everything she could to give me reassurance and show empathy. While she seemed sincere, I did have to wonder how many frightened patients had sat in this same room on this same bed, expressed the same fears and concerns, just to be told the exact same things. The fact of the matter was, there was no guarantee about how this was all going to pan out and my surgeon had been honest enough to tell me that.

After some time, they went out to the waiting room and invited my wife to join the conversation. Joanne told me about a couple things I'd have to do prior to surgery. The first, starting six days before The Day, was to take this medication called amiodarone. She didn't tell me at the time, but this stuff is normally used only to treat life-threatening heart rhythm disorders like ventricular tachycardia or ventricular fibrillation. There's all kinds of side effects to this drug including blurred vision, dizziness, gastrointestinal issues, irregular heartbeat, easy bruising/bleeding, loss of coordination, tingling/numbness of the hands or feet, fainting and uncontrolled movements. A nice little checklist. I'm telling you, these laboratory concocted drugs. So I hoped and prayed they'd not ask me to continue it after this was all over.

The second drug was this special mouth wash called chlorhexidine gluconate that I was to start taking three days prior. This also has fun side effects, though not as serious, including stained teeth and a messed-up sense of taste. They'd made a big deal about going to the dentist and making sure everything was good in my mouth as infections have been known to travel down to the heart arteries and cause major problems, if not death. I would later find out that this happened to a co-worker of mine and it led to a cardiac arrest. This mouth wash was to give my mouth and throat one final disinfectant cleansing and, I was told, could even help prevent me from inhaling bad things into my lungs. Powerful stuff.

The third was this special anti-bacterial soap I was to use for the final two showers before coming in, typically the night before and the morning of. I was given this small blue bottle and the instructions were to pour half of it on a washcloth and thoroughly scrub my chest and groin areas, then stand there and wait five minutes. After that I could rinse it off.

And whatever I did, I was *not* to attempt to shave my own chest or anything like that, because if there was even the slightest nick, the surgery may be postponed. Like Nora, my angiogram nurse, they'd do the shaving.

Oh, and don't even think about eating after midnight the night before. I'd expected that one.

The rest of my session with Joanne was just answering the usual questions about my overall health and habits. I'd had this same conversation with everyone recently, it seemed, but she dutifully documented everything in my record on the workstation. After that, like the anesthesiologist, she listened to my heart and lungs.

As she was tapping away at the computer, she said she just noticed that I'd not done my carotid ultrasound yet (that's where they do a sonagram of your neck to look at your arteries). Why not? Oh yeah, I'd heard about this from a message I'd gotten from someone at some point two or three weeks ago. I'd called back and they had no appointments available before the surgery date, so I dismissed it. But my surgeon had ordered it and wanted to see it before he started cutting. So apparently, it was a big deal. Joanne said she'd go find someone named Renee who could take care of this. She said they might be able to do it here today, but it would be a wait as they were pretty busy. Darn, I'd been looking forward to getting out early and having lunch with my wife in the city.

On the way out she gave me a sympathetic rub on the shoulder and a look that said, *just relax, everything is going to be fine.* Although that's what her expression conveyed, her actual words were, "Good luck with everything." *Right. Thanks.*

At this point I would have actually laughed if someone had said, *yeah, you might die, but we'll do our best.*

I saw an interview with David Letterman that had been taped few months after his quintuple coronary bypass surgery. His recovery had gone well and after just five weeks he had been back on TV hosting his program. But what struck me was how he'd said the whole event had been "so exciting." He did say though that "the rough part" was waking up with the breathing tube down your throat. I was seriously not looking forward to that.

A few minutes later I got my final visitor for that day, a nurse named Terry, whose job was to give me and my wife all the logistics of surgery day and the days to follow. Terry was high energy and spoke with intensity and passion, wide-eyed at times. She, like the others, clearly gave this speech and instructions to numerous patients, yet still seemed to really enjoy the purpose of her job.

On the morning of, I was to park at this address and then go to that address and check in at this time and so on. She gave me a bunch of information papers. I'd have to walk a block and half to the hospital. One of the many problems with San Francisco is limited space so things tend to be spread out. My check-in time, by the way, was 5:00 AM. Preparation was two hours, and the surgery was scheduled to start at 7:00.

Now, it may seem awful having a check-in time that early, but there are some real advantages. The first is that since I was Number One in line that day, the only thing that might cause delays would be if my surgeon or team members were needed for an unexpected emergency. It is, after all, a hospital where they do this kind of life-saving thing, so you never know. Second, assuming things went as planned and I was pulled out of general anesthesia at a normal time, I would not have to wait as long to get something to eat, assuming I could. Many are sick to their stomachs after anesthesia and throw up for awhile, but there were medications for that. There were meds for everything. I'd also been told you can feel really thirsty after this from the breathing tube air. So I didn't mind getting up early and getting this over with. I did feel for my wife though who'd be driving me.

Terry went on to explain the whole process of what's going to happen at the hospital, how'd I'd be taken out of bed and made to walk, a lot. My sleep would be totally disrupted as I'd get waken up, a lot, so that my vitals and other things could be checked. Much of this I knew from watching videos and reading stories. I felt a deep gratitude at that moment to the many people who've video-documented what they went through and posted it on YouTube and other places. It had given me a lot to learn and what to expect.

Terry also went into what she's seen and heard heart patients talk about. She emphasized, *you won't remember a thing*, assuring me that the actual surgery was "the easiest part." She also said that most don't even talk about the breathing tube because you're in a daze and won't remember much, just the last few minutes before they remove it. This kind of made me feel better, but again, my own research had tainted me.

Naturally, I'd watched a few videos on the whole extubating thing, and while some choke and have some difficulty, it looked pretty quick and fairly easy to most. One young guy though talked about how he'd gagged on the tube and accidentally bit his upper lip, causing it to swell. There's tests the nurses put you through to make sure you're conscious enough to be able to breath on your own. They make you look up at them and respond to questions or make hand gestures and such. If you pass, the tube gets removed. Oh boy, I couldn't wait.

And surprisingly, according to Terry, most don't even talk about the pain of the incision due to all the meds you're given. At least not while at the hospital. Its chest muscle pain and fatigue that many speak of. Finally, if all went well— meaning no complications and nothing unexpected—and I did my walking and breathing exercises, I might be discharged in as little as five days. Hopefully. Maybe…

Terry continued with what I was supposed to do and not do at home. Many of these instructions were directed at my wife. Don't even think about driving, and when I get driven by someone else, sit in the back seat as airbags were a no-no. Don't lift anything over ten pounds. Here's how the Tylenol plus codeine might make you feel. Have pets? Don't let them sit on you or put any weight on you. Here's a chart—fill out your daily weight, blood pressure and walking exercises and so on. I was also going to be visited by a nurse who does house calls the first week or two to see how you're doing. I hadn't been expecting that and didn't mind the news.

During our talk, the woman named Renee came by and said she found an appointment for my carotid ultrasound in Walnut Creek (CA) at 3:30 next Friday, could I make it? Yes, I could, thank you. So I'd have one more thing to do as it turned out. Okay, I'd deal with it.

Terry wrapped things up with a smile and a "good luck!" and I was sent on my way. As usual, she was careful not to guarantee me that everything was going to be just fine. Before leaving, I had to go back down to the sixth floor where a small pharmacy was to pick up the heart rhythm drug and mouthwash.

It was close to lunch and we'd be able find something to eat before going home. I walked out with the bag of drugs thinking, *Well, no turning back now…*

The Carotid Ultrasound

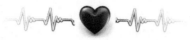

"Blood vessels are not cleaned with blood."

—Georgian Proverb

A s mentioned, there was one remaining procedure that had to be done and they weren't going to let me get away with not doing it prior to surgery. It's called a *carotid ultrasound*, also called an *ultrasonography*.

Similar to an echocardiogram, the procedure is a non-invasive, ultrasound-based diagnostic imaging technique to reveal structural details of the carotid arteries. These rather important tubes, connected directly to the aorta, feed the brain with fresh blood. While peering into one's neck, they look for blood clots, atherosclerotic plaque buildup, and anything else that may thwart blood flow.

The carotid arteries, two of them, a left and a right, jut out of the aortic arch portion, the crest of the "candy cane," and carry oxygenated blood to the neck and head. For whatever reason, most people are more familiar with the jugular veins which are close by and carry the blood already used by the brain back down the neck. Maybe the word "jugular" just sounds cooler.

On the drive over to Walnut Creek, I thought about another uncle of mine—a different one, not the one who had had the open-heart surgery and resulting stroke. This uncle had been a smoker and heavy drinker for almost 50 years and died a rather unpleasant death from various complications caused by alcoholism. But he'd been close to dying for a while for another reason—his carotid arteries were clogged up with tar and gunk from all that smoking he did. I don't think he had had a very healthy diet either, although he was never obese. At one point, he had tried desperately to quit smoking—the patch, various therapies, even hypnosis, but could not quit. Doctors had warned him that at "any time," pieces of this stuff in his arteries could break off, go to his brain, and cause a massive stroke. I was assuming they'd made that discovery via a carotid ultrasound, though I am not sure.

I myself smoked for five or six years between high school and college, and at that moment was sure glad I'd quit when I did. The famed trumpeter, Miles Davis, once said that out of all the stuff he had to stop doing, which included alcohol and heroin, smoking had been the hardest. And I believe it. It took me three tries and almost going insane, but finally succeeded, and that was after only five or six years. I can't imagine trying to quit after five or six decades.

Anyway, when I arrived at the hospital, I was told to go to the "vascular surgery" department on the third floor. When I checked in at the desk, I was actually directed to an area that had "Plastic Surgery" signs. Nice.

To distract myself, I waited near a section geared for occupying children and read a book about an octopus navigating the ocean floor, trying to avoid danger as it looked for a home. At one point it used its ink as camouflage to get away from a hungry moray eel. Isn't that the way of all the living, avoiding danger and just trying to live? The illustrations were very good; I admired the artist. You remember odd moments like this when your mind and body are under stress.

After a few minutes, my name was called by a guy in scrubs who introduced himself as "Chris". He was in his early to mid-50's maybe, and didn't have the authoritative air of a doctor or nurse, so I figured he was a technician of sorts.

I was led to a room that was similar to the echocardiogram setting. It had a bed, a few chairs and a desk, and some hampers with "used linen," "waste," and other signs. Chris told me this would be quick and painless and to go ahead and lie down on the bed. He had a calm and pleasant way about him. He also smiled easily, but didn't smile "too much" just for the sake of it, the way many do. I liked him already.

When I laid down, he turned a few lights off and the room became darker, but not as dark as when I had had the echocardiogram. He pulled a console on wheels over next to the bed with a setup that was just like the echo—the monitor with the keys and buttons and rollerball. He told me to turn my head to the left. After tucking a small face towel into my shirt like a bib, he took this tube which looked like a hand lotion product and squeezed out this goopy stuff directly on my neck. I'm guessing it was the same or similar stuff used for echos. It wasn't cold or unpleasant, just room temperature.

The magic wand/transducer was then placed on my neck and the images immediately appeared on the monitor. I couldn't see much yet because I was turned the other way, but they looked very similar to the echocardiogram in terms of the grainy, silver-white on black background.

But now, instead of the chambers and moving valves of my heart, it was the inside of my neck.

For the next five to seven minutes, Chris moved the wand just a little up and down while capturing images. He had a very gentle touch; the wand's end wasn't pressed up hard against me like the way they'd had done it during the echo. He also cranked up the volume at one point and I heard that distinct swishing, swirling sound of blood getting pumped through my arteries. These sounds of life we normally don't hear are always a little wow-inspiring. They are to me, anyway. You'd think your ear drums could pick up this stuff, but I guess we're wired to ignore those internal sounds.

"Well, this side passes with flying colors," Chris announced after a few minutes, referring to the right side of my neck. "No problems." That was good to hear.

I was asked to turn to my right and now I could see the monitor a lot better. Chris applied the goop again and started the same procedure, this time to the left side of my neck. I stared at the monitor, looking at the lines and tubes that were the blood hoses in my neck. They vaguely looked like close-ups of a section of a tree's root system. It also reminded me of when I was a kid and got an ant farm kit. It fascinated me to watch the ants dig a tunnel system in the dirt packed in the narrow space between the glass walls.

The next image is a still from my ultrasonography session with Chris.

Video still image: Carotid ultrasound

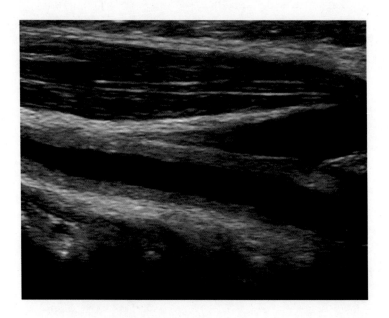

Image source: Kelly Libatique (n.d.). No copyright.

Just for conversation, I guess, Chris asked me what this was for and I told him about my upcoming open-heart surgery. To my relief, he didn't flinch, didn't say, "Oh, I'm sorry to hear that" or give me an, *I pity you* look. He just continued and asked if it was Dr. So and So (Dr. Dan, my surgeon) and I said yes. Chris said they do five or six of these carotid ultrasounds a week just for them—the surgery team in San Francisco—and that they are "a busy crew."

Once again, I was a little surprised to hear how many people have problems in the area of cardiovascular disease. Heart disease is, in fact, the number one cause of early or preventable death in America, I would find out. Sitting around in front of computers with our slick, convenient technology apparently hasn't been too healthy for us as a society. Add to that the superficial and plastic nature of our online social media interactions and it's clear we're doing ourselves more harm than good. But then again, I don't use social media myself and look what happened to me.

I glanced up at a certificate in a frame on the wall and saw that it said something about Christopher so and so being a certified sonographer. There was my answer as to what he was.

After just a few more minutes we wrapped up and I was given a towel to clean the goop off my neck. Chris told me everything looks great and I've no issues. One more bullet dodged. *Whew…*

I asked Chris if the machine was the same used in echocardiograms and he said it was almost the same but that the software was a little different. I then asked where one goes to school to become a certified sonographer, I was just curious. He told me that back in the 80's when he did it, it had been up in Washington. At the time, he said, there were only three schools in the country that gave the certi-fication, but there were a lot more now. He went on to say there were a bunch of prerequisites like anatomy classes and such one had to take, which made sense.

I walked away feeling a sense of relief but also knowing that I was close to the one-week countdown until surgery.

Time was a-flyin'.

The Operation

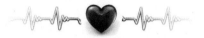

**"Sometimes the people around you won't
understand your journey. And that's okay.
They don't need to. It's not for them."**

—Unknown

Before going into what happened the morning of
The Day, I want to first mention something briefly
about scheduling the operation. At some point after
the initial face-to-face with your surgeon, you're going to
need to schedule when it's going to happen. Doctors and
hospitals are busy, and you need to get in line, typically.

I've been in countries where people routinely have to
wait months or even over a year for these procedures, but
that wouldn't be the case with me. I may not have survived
that, who knows. I would schedule mine in early October, a
week or so before the coronary angiogram. From there, I'd
end up only having about two weeks to wait.

Someone from the hospital's "scheduling office" had
called and left a message on my phone, and I remember a
strange feeling come over me as I listened to the message.
The woman leaving it could have been calling from the dry
cleaners. The language was the usual, *Hi, this is so and so
from Dr. so and so's office, I'd like to talk to you about a surgery*

date…She didn't say it in an indifferent or uncaring way, she just said it so…business as usual-like. The same kind of casualty that I'd sensed from my surgeon. That icky sense of, *don't you know I'm a scared, unique human being instead of surgery patient number 499 for the year?*, was cropping up again. But really, what did I expect? Did I want people to coddle and talk to me like a lost child at the mall? Apparently, a part of me who was, indeed, a scared little kid, did. Remember, this is the first time I'd been through anything like this. Everything about this was making me anxious. But to these folks, it was just their job. Besides, they knew they were talking to someone who was almost 50. I needed to stop being juvenile and push these feelings aside.

So I called back and found that bookings were in short order and the rest of the year was getting filled up fast. Wow, that many people needed surgery. The heart murmur in my chest had been discovered in late August, the tests done September through mid-October, and the next available surgery date was November 4. I'm guessing most avoid surgeries in December unless it's urgent, of course. I certainly wouldn't want to be stuck in the hospital during Christmas as many are.

I ended up booking it for a Monday, November 4—and there it was, an actual date. If the reality of your situation hadn't settled in by now, it will once you've got a date. Friends and family want to know, of course, and now you can tell them. And when you tell people, it's a weird feeling too. Like there's no backing out now. I had a wall calendar at my work office and I'd stare at that date and know how fast it's going to come. There was no wishing time would slow or stop to avoid the inevitable. The weeks were moving at an appalling speed.

The day before this, I'd had my wife take one last picture of my chest so it would be documented how it looked before all this. It sounds silly, I know. But I knew I'd never be the same. God had given me this one and only body and people were going to swap some parts and make permanent changes.

Well, the morning of The Day came. I'd say it came "at last," but this whole thing had leapt upon me like an ambush predator. Well, not quite true—you don't see predators coming, not the skilled ones anyway. I'd been dutifully taking my heart rhythm drug amiodarone for the last six days and I was feeling some of its effects. I was really tired of the low circulation, lack of energy, slightly dizzy and cold hands this drug was causing.

I had gotten maybe two hours of sleep the night before, not because I drifted off peacefully, but more like passed out from exhaustion. I suppose I should be grateful I got at least that. But lying there awake anticipating the next morning was no fun, and it was impossible to clear my mind.

At around 3:30 am, I got up and took my final shower. I scrubbed myself and hair hard as I knew I may not be getting another shower for several days. I used the last of the anti-bacterial soap they'd given me and stared at my chest as I rubbed it in. It would never look the same again. There'd be a big scar running the length of my sternum as well as a couple holes below it for drainage tubes. It wasn't that my aspirations of being a swimsuit model were being destroyed, it was just a weird feeling that my body will be forever changed for the remainder of my time in this life.

After putting on the most comfortable clothes I had, an old pair of jogging pants, a t-shirt, and sweat jacket, we shuffled out the door. It was about 4:00 AM and I got into the car with my wife. She volunteered to drive. A feeling of apprehension was riveting through me, the likes of which I'd never felt before. The air outside was crisp, chilly, and the sky still dark. It was still. No wind.

We drove in silence. I didn't want to talk, didn't want to listen to music. This day had come so fast it'd made my head spin. As I'd mentioned, for the last several weeks, I'd been staring at a calendar. With each appointment, each test, whatever I had to do, I'd watch the days whir by. During the final week, I just wanted to do this and get it over with. I was tired of waiting and tired of learning more about human anatomy. I didn't want to watch any more videos on other people's experiences. I just wanted to wake up and know I'd made it through without complications or unexpected surprises.

I tried to make myself feel better by thinking of funny things. One of my favorite comedians, Rodney Dangerfield once said, "I asked the doctor how long am I going to be in the hospital? He said, if all goes well, about a week…if it doesn't, about 30 minutes." I smirked, but then thought about the fact that Rodney had passed away after heart surgery. He was 82 though and I was much younger.

We arrived at the parking garage about 15 minutes before check-in time which was perfect. I didn't bring a bag or anything with me. In case things went south, I was just going to give everything like my wallet and cellphone to my wife to hang on to. And like with the MRI session, I'd left my wedding ring at home. I was going to walk into this with just the clothes on my back and then hopefully walk out the same way.

We sat in the waiting room as usual. I could have been there waiting for the usual checkup, but this time it was different. The place was very quiet, no one else there this time of morning. I kind of liked that. No one hurrying around or acting uptight. With the exception of one other quiet couple in the corner, I had the place all to myself at that moment.

A guy behind a desk had me sign in and told me someone would be with me shortly. I sat and looked around at the generic pictures on the wall, the computer screens, the hand sanitizer stations. I imagined my surgeon, anesthesiologist and other operating room staff getting up and going about their morning routine. For them, it was just another Monday, another set of patients. For me, it was a make it or break it day, a day that, if I survived, would change my life forever.

I momentarily watched the couple in the corner and could tell by the body language that, like me, it was the guy who was the patient today. He would lean forward with his face in his hands and she would rub his back in a soothing manner. I wondered how many *everything's going to be okay, honey* scenarios played out each week in this very room.

As we waited, two more couples came in, both 15 to 20 years older than myself. After a few more minutes, a final couple came in and as they walked across the room, the lady looked at all of us and said, "You too, huh?"

For a brief moment, the heavy atmosphere in the room was lightened by a little laughter.

A woman finally came in and went across the room and opened an office. We all stared at her in silence and she didn't acknowledge any of us. Just another early morning check-in crowd. After a couple minutes she called the first couple in that I'd seen in the beginning. The office door was shut and I watched them through the glass.

After about ten minutes, it was my turn. I was asked if I'd seen the standard consent form before, which I had from the coronary angiogram appointment. I signed it, paid my insurance co-pay, and was assigned a patient number. I imagined that number as a tag on a body bag in a few hours. *Stop, it okay?* I was then was instructed to go to the next floor up to a certain waiting room adjacent to this big prep area.

In the next 30 minutes or so, all the couples I'd seen in the registration waiting room came into this same waiting room. We were all there for early morning surgery, or half of us anyway. The other half were there for support. We were a quiet bunch, and the air was thick with tension and apprehension. Except for one smiley guy who, honest to God, almost seemed to be having a good time.

At some point, my wife wandered over to this flat screen on the wall that showed the status of the patients: pre-surgery, during surgery, post-surgery, and so on. For privacy, the screen displayed no names, only numbers. The couple with the smiley guy was there and my wife got into a conversation with them. Apparently, this guy had been through three or four other surgeries and wasn't worried. Or at least he wasn't showing any worry. When my wife returned, she tried to assure me by telling me his story.

At last a nurse called my name and my wife accompanied me while I followed the nurse to this prep room. It was just another curtained off section of a larger room with a bed and equipment. I was told to undress and put on the usual hospital gown. After taking all my vitals and asking a bunch of questions, the nurse stuck what could be best described as a giant, dinner plate-sized band aid on my butt. I was told that because of the length of time I'd be lying in bed, this was to protect me from bedsores. She also put one of those IVs with the short tube into my arm which would stay for the remainder of my stay at the hospital.

During this time a young guy, late 20's, came in and introduced himself as the one who was going to shave me. It would be like what Nora had done to me before the angiogram, but a lot more. He was going to shave me clean "from the knees up." Nice.

I was watching the clock and we were maybe 40 minutes or so from the 7:00 AM scheduled start time of the surgery when I was told to lay on the bed and get ready to be moved. My wife was invited to follow as I was wheeled down a series of halls to another large room with curtain-separated areas. This place was bustling with nurses and technicians who were running around doing the final preparations for people going into various surgical procedures.

After I was parked in my curtained stall, a guy in his mid-30's introduced himself as Joey and began looking me over. He kept asking if I had any questions and was speaking in a well-trained way to sound comforting and reassuring. I wasn't acting scared or saying anything negative, at least not that I was aware of. I didn't want to bother with any of that nonsense. The time had come and honestly, I didn't feel all that frightened. Or maybe I was in a little shock and just didn't have the energy anymore to entertain fear. Sure, I still had some apprehension, but I certainly wasn't wide-eyes and shaking.

Some worker came in with a clipboard and started asking questions. One of them was a final confirmation that I had chosen a tissue/bioprosthetic valve as the one to replace my native aortic valve. I confidently said yes, though inside

I felt anything but confidence. She marked down all my answers and then left.

The young guy who was going to shave me came in with this special looking electric shaver and started carefully adjusting my gown so he could get to all the places he needed to.

While he was shaving, I asked him how many people he shaves here each week and he said, "Oh, a lot."

I asked, "The women too?" He said yes.

"Do they object to this?" I asked.

He just smiled and said, "Some do."

The room temperature was the usual hospital-cold and at some point, Joey stuck a hose under the thin blanket that was over me that started blowing warm air. It felt pretty good, actually.

The next picture shows me in the prep room just a few minutes before surgery. I don't look scared...do I?

Photo: In the prep room right before surgery

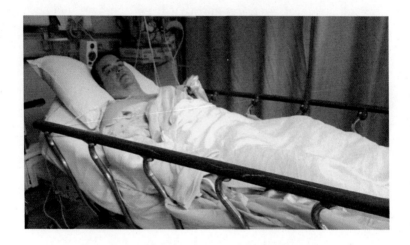

Image source: Kelly Libatique (n.d.). No copyright

Finally, my assigned anesthesiologist came by and introduced herself. Dr. So and So had told me during the pre-op that it may not be him that morning, and it wasn't. It was a young, cheerful woman, early to mid-30's, short, curly blonde hair, with a pleasant smile and demeanor. She introduced herself and I honestly don't remember the name, probably because I was thinking about some questions I wanted to ask and I was distracted by the guy shaving me. She briefly explained what she was going to do, that I will not be aware of anything and that it will be over quickly, and so on.

Then I asked her, "Anesthesia awareness has never happened here, right?"

She said, "In my eight years here, I've never heard of it happening, no." I can read people pretty well, and I believed her.

"While preparing for all this, I did some exercises in mental masochism and researched this and it scared me pretty good. So I had to ask," I said.

She smiled and said, "Totally fair." Then she said goodbye and left.

I looked up at the clock and it was 6:45 - 15 minutes to show time. And then something totally unexpected happened. Out of the blue, Dr. Dan, my surgeon, suddenly popped through the curtain and came to the side of my bed. He asked how I was doing and I bravely said I was doing fine.

Then he took hold of the bed rails, leaned in and looked at me urgently. "I know you wanted a tissue valve, but I really don't want to do that," he said.

What?!

154

My mind reeled. I may have said, *Uhm, okay,* but I really don't remember. Or I may have just stared at him in dazed disbelief because he continued.

"If we give you a tissue valve, at your age, it's going to wear out in five or ten years and we'll have to go in again and replace it. You wouldn't want to go through this surgery again. I think we should go with a mechanical valve."

I took note of the word *we.* Was this some psychological trick? Like, *you and me, we're in this together,* kind of thing? This was my heart, not his…

I may have said, *you're right, I wouldn't want to do that.* But I think I was slipping back into a little shock because I do remember just staring again, waiting, I guess, for more explanation, although more was probably not needed.

"When the valve needs replacing," Dr. Dan continued, "we won't be able to go in with a catheter procedure. This is because of the aneurism that needs replacing. That would mess up the graft and all that we're going to do there. We would have to open you up again, stop everything [meaning shut down my heart again] and that wouldn't be worth the risk."

I have to admit I was impressed he'd remembered details of our conversation from weeks ago and wondered how many other patients he'd spoken to since. Well, people with poor memories don't become surgeons, do they. During our talk a few weeks ago, I had mentioned that if I did the tissue valve, I thought that any procedure going forward could be done with all this cool new technology that was available with transcatheter stuff. But that was an assumption and a gamble not worth taking, in Dr. Dan's opinion.

"You don't want to do that again ten years from now," he said, reiterating the thought and now talking more like he was giving a hard sale.

I had one last chance to be cynical and desperate about my situation, so I said, "Well, if I'm even still around in ten years."

He looked firmly at me and said, "Oh you'll still be here in ten years."

Later, when I'd thought about that moment, I realized it was an asinine thing to say and I regret it. Here he was an experienced surgeon with 27 years under his belt. I may have been the 3,000th patient he'd operated on, but yet here he was looking out for what I believe he thought were my best interests. If he didn't care, he could have not bothered coming to me last minute and having this conversation. I should have been grateful, but I was being driven by a lot of loud emotions.

He was still staring at me and started to say something else, but I held up a hand and said, "It's okay, you've sold me." Then in my mind I thought to myself, *Well, after all your anti-Coumadin ranting, you just committed yourself to taking the stuff for life.*

He nodded and quietly said, "Okay." I know I made the *sold me* comment with no smile and probably a regretful look in my eyes. Maybe he wasn't sure what else to say. He gave me an assuring nod and turned to leave.

My wife would later tell me that she had been listening to this conversation and praying that I'd say yes to the mechanical valve. She knew I didn't want to take anti-co-agulant drugs the rest of my life. But she, like Dr. Dan, wanted what was best for me long term. Her prayers had been answered.

A couple minutes after 7:00 and it was time to go. My wife was told that this was where she had to leave to return to the waiting room. There were several places she could go. There were rooms right next to the operating rooms where there was space for five or six. Some like to be physical close in proximity to where their loved ones are under the knife. But my wife went downstairs to meet my brother and mom who had also come along to add their support.

A large, stocky man in his mid to late 30's with a thick Kenyon accent began wheeling my bed down the hall to the operating room. We stopped by the door and he looked through a small window, waiting to be beckoned by the surgical team.

I asked him how many heart patients he wheels around here each week and he said, "Oh lots. Many patients."

I told him there must be something wrong with our culture or society for there to be that many people who need procedures done to their hearts. We got into a little conversation about how all our technology and social media and everything else is apparently not very healthy.

Then he said something about my situation I'll not forget. He made the comment, "In Africa, you would just die. You would have no help."

It gave me pause. Here I'd been pouting about life's circumstances when I could be where there were no hospitals ready to do open-heart surgery and experienced doctors and staff who knew how to do it. I've travelled around parts of Asia and the Middle East and it's true that unless you're one of the rich who could be quickly carted off to some place where this stuff was done, *you'd* be done. I will never forget that moment.

At last he was given the signal and I was wheeled into the operating room. Because I was lying flat on my back I wasn't able to see a lot, but it was definitely a classic room where major surgery is performed.

My mobile bed was moved alongside the main bed and I was asked to scoot myself over to it. I did, and after adjusting, an object was placed under my shoulder blades that felt like a firm, tube-shaped pillow that kept my chest raised up. Someone in the room told me that it might be a little uncomfortable, but it was needed.

I laid there on the table staring up at the bright, round lights on the ceiling you only see in operating rooms. I could have looked around a little more but just didn't want to. I only stared at the light wondering what going under was going to feel like.

Did I really volunteer for this? I asked myself. *Yes, but was I given a choice?* Sort of, maybe. I thought I was going to see the anesthesiologist put the mask over my nose or something like that, but I didn't. I thought maybe I'd see a cloud of blackness close in over my vision. But all I remember seeing was the lights and a few people milling around in my peripheral vision. They must have hooked something up to the IV in my arm because the next thing I knew, it was over.

The next photo I had to throw in here, even though I didn't see a bunch of people all staring at me like that. I did see those big round lights though and staff bustling about me in my peripheral vision. It's an intimidating moment.

Photo: On the operating table

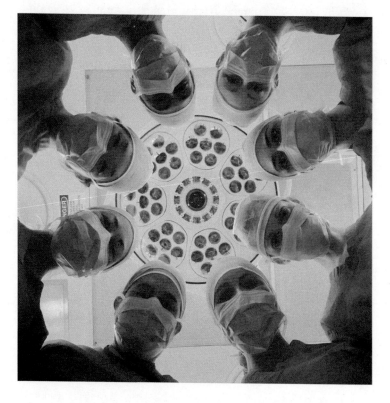

Photo by the National Cancer Institute (Jun 7, 2020) on Unsplash.
Retrieved from https://unsplash.com/photos/701-FJcjLAQ

The next thing I knew, it was over. It's very strange to come out of general anesthesia when you have no recollection of going into it. I remember "seeing" a wall of blackness and then heard voices. I was aware that some time had passed but I couldn't tell how much. If I had to guess, I might have said maybe 20 minutes had gone by. In reality, I'd been out for almost seven and half hours.

I'd find out later that the operation lasted about five hours, from 7:00 AM to noon. But then they kept me under for another two and a half hours or so in case something went wrong and they had to rush me back into the operating room. I had been told during the pre-op that this was standard operating procedure, so it was of no surprise.

I also found out later that my wife, mother and brother, his wife, and a friend had been allowed into the recovery room in ICU after the doctors and nurses ensured I was stable. They had been there at my bedside watching me while I was out and with that breathing tube down my throat. My wife was going to take a picture of me, but the nurse told her not to unless I'd given permission, so she did not. That's actually kind of nice of them, but I would have given permission as I'd be curious to know how I looked. My mother later commented that I looked "peaceful."

By the time I was coming to, my family was already gone. The voices I heard were that of nurses and whoever else was in the room. The wall of blackness melted away as I struggled to open my eyes and blink.

Now, I'd seen videos of people coming out of general anesthesia and that stuff can make people a mess. Some babbling, some cussing, some confessing sins, some falling in love with and proposing to hospital staff. All kinds of things. So before I went under, or the day before, I'd prayed that when I came out of my chemically induced coma, I'd not be like that. Especially if family and friends were around. And my prayers were answered. When I finally got my vision, I immediately knew exactly where I was and what had happened to me.

I remember seeing at least two people staring at me and felt the breathing tube. This was another thing that had scared me—having a big tube shoved down my throat. But it wasn't painful at all, nor was it making me choke and gag. The tube was small in diameter, no more than a straw. It reminded me of an aquarium air pump tube. But I could feel the little ballooned portion deep down in my throat, somewhere near my trachea, that was keeping it wedged and unmoving. I could also feel the strange sensation of the machine pushing air into my lungs, then drawing it back out again.

One of the nurses may have said something along the lines of, *there he is* or *he's coming to*, but it's hard to remember. The drugs were still potent in me and I wasn't sure what I was feeling.

After a minute or two, one of the nurses took my right hand and asked, "Can you squeeze my hand?" I squeezed twice.

The other nurse took my left hand and said, "Can you squeeze this hand?" I obliged.

Then one of them asked, "Can you wiggle your toes?" I felt one of them put her hand on my toes and I wiggled them as best as I could.

Apparently satisfied with my responses, one of them said something about *okay, we can remove this*, referring to the breathing tube. I remember thinking I should be nervous, but I guess I was too drugged up to care much. They pulled my jaw down a little and commented that some of the tube had gotten bunched up in my mouth. I hadn't noticed. I was told to get ready to cough, which seemed a bit impossible, but I'd try. One of the nurses started pulling the tube and I managed a couple weak coughs. The next thing I knew, the tube was out and I could breathe on my own. It was quick and painless, and I never gagged or choked.

I sucked air in and out as best as I could and looked around. The room I was in was still in ICU, but it didn't look like anything unusual. My breaths were very shallow and my chest felt tight and heavy, but otherwise there was no pain of any kind. Not yet.

I tried to relax and get my head wrapped around what I'd just been through. I'd survived. I'd not woken up in eternity. My physical body, albeit now permanently changed, was still here. I was a living patient, not a number on a bag downstairs in the morgue. So much of what I'd feared and anticipated had not happened. Wow.

But what was to come now?

Recovery in the Hospital

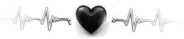

"It feels good to hear someone say *take care*, but it feels so much better to hear, *I will take care of you*."

—Unknown

In the world of surgery, they consider "Day 1" the next day after surgery, but I kind of feel like day one was the actual day *of.*

It had maybe been an hour or two after I'd come out of general anesthesia and I was being introduced to several individuals. Most of them were nurses or staff in ICU and one of them was a physical therapist. The therapist was a woman in her late 20's or early 30's who had a stern, humorless way about her. We'd get along just fine.

I knew from watching videos of other's experiences that they were going to force me to move at least somewhat on the day of surgery. Apparently, moving and getting one's circulation going is key to recovery, and I didn't want to spend more time in the hospital than I needed to.

It took a while to grasp what they'd done to me. First, there was a long incision line running the length of my sternum bone from top to bottom. It was bright red and swollen around the edges and looked pretty nasty. In addition to dissolvable stiches (made from either chemical sugars or collagen from animals, I didn't know which were mine), there was a glue applied over the incision that sort of resembled silicon. My sternum bone underneath I knew was being held together with wires made from either titanium or stainless steel. These would be in me for life, unless complications arose.

The next image shows an x-ray of my chest a couple days after surgery. Those zigzagging, crisscrossing lines down my sternum are one of the new permanent accessories in my body. It'll be interesting the first time I go through an airport x-ray machine with these—the place will probably light up like a pinball machine.

Image: X-ray of sternum wires

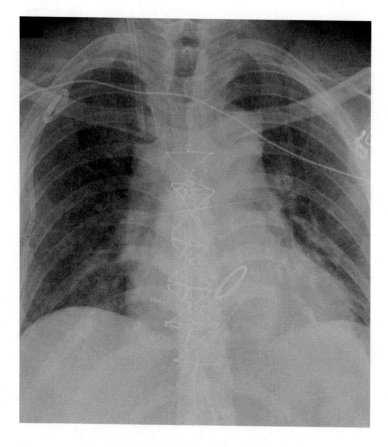

Image source: Kelly Libatique (n.d.). No copyright

But the incision down my sternum was nothing compared to the three tubes hanging out from me directly below the incision. They were covered by and protruding out from under a large bandage. Although I felt nothing yet, they would prove to be quite uncomfortable. These tubes are for draining fluids that build up around and under one's heart following surgery of this type. They were connected to two different boxes on the floor that uses water suction to help pull the fluids down the tubes. The sound of it gurgling away reminded me of an aquarium filter.

There was more stuff in and on me I was too drugged up to notice yet. There were two wires above the tube incision that went up inside me and were actually touching my heart. These, apparently, are for the unfortunate folks who have heart attacks following surgery and need to be jump started. Makes sense—why not have the jumper cables in place, ready to go?

There were also three or four EKG electrode stickers next to the wire holes that were attached to a little portable device that was roughly the size of a walkie-talkie. I would have to carry this thing in the pocket of my hospital gown the entire time. This device sent a radio signal to something, somewhere, telling them how my heart was beating and such. With all this stuff hanging out of and off your body, you feel quite restrained and cannot do much of anything without help.

I also, at some point, became aware that my legs were getting massaged. After I went under, they'd wrapped these things around the lower parts of my legs that were gently massaging my calves. It would start from the top and work its way down. This, apparently, helps keep a little circulation going in your legs. It felt kind of good.

The physical therapist was asking if I could sit up. Here's where I felt a bit of pride, despite the circumstances I was in. All the sit-ups and squats I'd done at home in the weeks leading up to surgery was now paying off. I closed my eyes, squinted, and then pulled myself up.

The physical therapist commented, "You have a strong core. Very good."

After sitting up, I was instructed to wiggle myself to the edge of the bed, which I was able to do. I felt a bit queasy and dizzy, but otherwise okay. I took note that I didn't feel sick to my stomach. They kept asking how I was feeling and how much pain I was in and so forth, and I had to admit I was doing pretty good, all things considered.

Are you hungry? I was asked. This reminded me that I'd not had anything to eat since maybe 6:00 PM the night before, and here we were almost 12 hours later. I actually wasn't hungry, but maybe I'd try a little something. One of the nurses brought some broth in a little cup. It smelled good so I took a sip. Almost immediately, my stomach turned and I threw it up. It was a strange feeling. Normally, before throwing up, you feel that sickly sensation creeping up. But in this case, I didn't actually feel sick, I just could not hold anything down. No worries, this was all normal, I was assured.

In the weeks preceding all this, there was a video I saw of this young guy who needed heart surgery for some reason. He wasn't even 25 years old but had been born with a certain condition. But because of his age, he was up and about and eating full meals even on the day of surgery. Youth…I was disappointed I would not be able to eat like he had, but I was determined to show the nurses and staff, as well as myself, that I could move around.

Now it was time to try to stand up. A walker with wheels was brought over and the people around me carefully hung the gurgling boxes on bars at the bottom of the walker. With one person on each side of me, I was asked to slide off the bed and to my feet, which I was able to do fairly easily.

The physical therapist draped another gown over my back while saying, "No free shows here."

I smirked and said, "No one wants a free show from me." Nobody responded to the remark which led me to believe the *free shows* comment and my typical retort was an exchange made a dozen times a week there. Just another day in ICU for recovering heart patients.

Going by videos I'd seen of others, I began to march in place, even though the therapist had not asked me to do this. At least this would get my circulation going right away.

"Okay, let's do a little walking and see how far you get," the physical therapist said.

We slowly began out of the room. I felt dizzy and was now starting to feel a little nauseous, but I trudged on with determination. The therapist kept asking how I was feeling and I kept saying I'm okay even though I did have to lean a bit on the walker from the dizziness. But we made it around the block of that floor there and I was glad to get back into bed. I was told I did great.

I honestly don't remember a whole lot of surgery day, I guess because the general anesthesia was still doing its thing and you've got other pain killers in you to boot. I think I just laid down and went to sleep.

I don't really remember much about the next morning or how I slept either. I was seriously out of it. But when

I finally awoke and was more aware of my situation, it wasn't pleasant.

First off, you can hardly breathe. This kind of surgery leaves you with a feeling that a 300-pound person is standing on your chest. It's very difficult to inhale and it comes with a frustrating sensation that you can't get enough air.

They give you this little apparatus to use for breathing exercises, and it's not just to re-strengthen your lungs. After heart surgery, there's fluid buildup in your lungs which makes for a high risk getting pneumonia. The more and deeper you breathe, the more your lungs can "dry out," and the chances of pneumonia go down. The apparatus has a flexible tube with a mouthpiece connected to three joined plastic tubes with floating pieces that gauge how hard you can suck in air. The harder you inhale, the higher the plastic pieces rise in the tubes.

Then there is pain. Not only is it hard to breathe, it's painful as the drugs start to wear off. And here's the one big boon of having surgery like this: during the first three or so, they give you all the drugs you want.

Hospitals use a zero to ten system of pain. If you tell the staff you're feeling pain, they will ask you for the number representing your pain. Zero is no pain and ten is unbearable agony. If you say you're pain level is say, a three or a four, they'll give you large doses of acetaminophen. But if you're pain is a seven or eight or higher, they'll pull out the big guns and give you oxycodone, or oxytocin. One of those.

We've all heard about the ongoing opioid crisis and all the overdoses, and oxycodone is one of the main culprits. I can see why. That stuff works. At one point, I felt like I was gasping like a drowning person. The pressure on my chest was intense, and every time I inhaled it was hurting more. I told the nurse I was in pain and was asked to give a number. I said at least an eight. He disappeared and quickly reappeared with a syringe that was designed to inject into IVs. I watched as the clear liquid went into the contraption on my arm and within seconds felt its soothing effects. I'm not sure what the liquid was, but a warmness creeps up on you and brings sweet relief to any pains you may be feeling—"Comfortably Numb," like the title of the famous Pink Floyd song. It felt like my chest was being opened up, but in a good and comforting way.

On top of the injection, which brings immediate relief, they also give you a couple of tiny pills that act as longer-lasting relief. They take 15 to 20 minutes to kick in. After several times of the injection and pill routine, I'd watch the clock and anticipate the sweet sensation of having no pain at all, despite everything my body was enduring.

I remember this one time I was about to take the tiny pills, which are maybe the size of baby aspirin, when they fell out of my hand into the folds of the bed sheet, maybe on the floor. The nurse got a little nervous and said we need to find those, remarking that he'd have "a hard time explaining to his supervisor where some extra narcotics went." So, they have problems with drugs getting smuggled out of there too, eh? I didn't ask, but that was clearly the implication. The system that keeps track of all those patients must be pretty sophisticated. We found the pills, by the way.

One of the big side effects of this drug though is sleepiness. I can image, now, being hooked on this stuff and what it would do to you if you consumed it all the time. I slept constantly those first three days, whether I was in the bed or in the chair. And it was great. No matter what position I was in, dozing off was easy. If I requested to be moved to the chair, one or two nurses would move all my boxes and tubes to the right side of the bed and assist while I stood up and waddled to the chair. Once in the chair, I would lean my head forward and nod off again.

Besides the difficult breathing, I also temporarily lost my voice. As a voice-over talent, this kind of scared me—I depend on having a strong voice. But when I was alert enough to realize how I sounded, my voice was high-pitched, squeaky, and whispery. It would remain this way for my stay at the hospital and I seriously started to wonder if I'd ever sound the same. I would eventually get my voice back, but not until about three days after I'd returned home. When I called one of my doctors, she was shocked it was me because I sounded so different.

While I did sleep most of the time those first three days, sleeping uninterrupted for long periods is impossible. Every eight hours, around the clock, the new nurse for that shift would come in and the first thing they need to do is check your vitals and administer any needed drugs. The nurse named Terry at the pre-op had warned me about this. One of the shifts started at midnight. This means that every night at midnight I was awakened by a nurse wrapping a blood pressure cuff around my arm and sticking a thermometer in my mouth and asking me questions. I was annoyed but I didn't get mad at them, they were just doing their job.

The significance of getting woken up at all hours for me is my sleep apnea. I'd told them about it and so they had someone from their "respiratory team" bring a CPAP machine into the room. I was able to use it the first two nights but then I gave up. The problem was that it's hard to get back to sleep once I've been woken up. I wasn't tired enough to have it put on until around 9:00 PM, and then it took until close to 10:00 to finally fall asleep. Plus, I'm not used to having someone else put the mask on and then not having control to turn it on and off—the machine was located too far away for me to reach.

The first night I used the CPAP, I was so drugged up that after the nurse woke me up at midnight, I was actually able to drift back off again. It was great. Sometime that morning, maybe around 4:00 AM, I awoke and took the mask off which caused the machine to alarm. Eventually someone came in and turned the alarm off.

The second night, it took a long time to get back to sleep—almost two hours. You have to lie there helpless because again, I could not turn the machine off, and removing the mask caused an alarm. The third night I got woken up, I asked the nurse to just remove the mask entirely and turn the machine off. She apologized profusely for waking me up, but I told her not to worry about it. We were all doing what we needed to do. For the remainder of my time at the hospital, when someone from the respiratory team offered to put the CPAP mask on, I told them I wasn't going to bother using it.

Another routine that was tough was the daily blood draw. Each morning, around 8:00 maybe, this young guy from the lab would pay me a visit. He carried with him the usual implements for phlebotomy: the blood collection needles and tubes, the rubber elastic arm band, cotton ball and bandage and so on. He usually stuck me in the veins protruding from the back of my left hand. One morning, I think the fourth, he returned after a few minutes and nervously asked if he could draw blood again. He looked quite timid as he apologized up and down for having to do it again so soon. Out of curiosity, I asked if he'd not gotten enough. He said something about how he'd used the wrong collecting tube. I didn't get mad, I could tell he'd taken heat from patients before. I just held out my hand and let him do what he had to do.

The first day after surgery, or Day Two, came with another unpleasant surprise for me. A young female technician wheeled a portable x-ray machine in to take a picture of my chest. I was lying in bed at the time and very drugged up and watched sleepily as she draped the heavy lead-filled thing over my abdomen. A red "X" appeared on my chest as she adjusted and aimed the machine at me. A minute later it was over, and the contraption was wheeled away. But then an hour two later, after the doctors looked at the images, I got some bad news.

The surgery had caused my right lung to partially collapse. Uhm…what does that mean? Well, it explained in part why breathing was so difficult. But whatever else it indicated, it needed to be fixed. They felt I was too out of it to give permission to drill any more holes into me, so they asked my wife, and she said yes.

So in my dazed and confused state, they wheeled me back into a surgery room, not the same one that was used for the major surgery, but a smaller one. They did not put me under like with general anesthesia, but they must have given me a little more of something because I was pretty loopy, albeit conscious. I do remember a couple guys manhandling me from the mobile bed to another stationary one. I was then turned on my left side. I must have felt like a 200-pound sack of potatoes, but they seemed to be pretty used to it.

While on my side, someone started doing something to the right side of my chest. I felt it, but didn't want to look. I would later find out they'd cut another hole in me and put yet another tube similar to the three drainage tubes under my main chest incision. This tube went to my right lung and was attached to another box that was doing something to fix the collapsed part. So now I had a total of four tubes and three boxes hanging from my body. I felt like a freak version of Dr. Octavia from *Spiderman*.

When I try to remember those first three days, it's all pretty blurry. This is both the blessing and curse of powerful drugs. I would not have done it any different, meaning I'd take the drugs again, because those first days are pretty awful in terms of waking up with wires, stitches and tubes. At the same time though, you definitely want to just sleep through it as much as you can—between your walking exercises of course. If you don't get up and walk every day, your hospital stay is going to be longer.

You also feel weak, so much so you can do almost without great effort. I remember lying there thinking, a five-year-old could come in here and start beating me up and there wouldn't be a thing I could do about it. If the place caught on fire and no one wheeled me out, that'd be the end of me. You find out what the word *helpless* really means and it's humbling.

It was on the morning of the third day that I asked them to help me into the chair. They did, and I stayed there most of the day. It turns out that was a good thing because one's circulation is a little better sitting up then when lying down. Or so I was told. The problem was that the physical therapist had forgotten about me or was too busy and never came to visit. So I sat there for nearly the entire day watching the little television screen attached to the ceiling.

While I was in that chair, my wife and mother came to visit. I encourage all those reading this to visit someone you know in a hospital. It's a most welcome site. They came in with small plants they'd bought from someone on the street nearby and set them on the windowsill. For the rest of my stay, I would look at those little plants and think of the life they possess. After my stay, I'd take them home and re-plant them in a nice pot.

Another thing I remember was being cold all the time. I had heard my roommate complaining about that as well. The room always felt chilly. Turns out that after open-heart surgery, your circulation is bit messed up for awhile. No surprise. This would last the first couple weeks at home too. But no matter what position you're in, you feel like you want to wrap up in blankets. This makes the constant going to the bathroom from the all the diuretics they give you a challenge.

Now, sometime between the third and fourth day, they start easing you off the drugs. This is good in the sense that you don't want to become a narcotics addict. But it's bad in that the times they can administer the drugs start getting more spread out. The computer terminal the nurses use to do their routine tells them at exactly what time they can give you the next dose of this or that. If there's still 18 minutes to go before the next dose, you need to wait for those 18 minutes, no exceptions. The result is that sleeping becomes even more difficult. Without the same amount of drugs, you feel the pain and laborious breathing more. And if you have back problems like I do after lying in one position for a long time, those will keep you awake as well.

I had my first meal, I think, at lunch time during the third day. They were starting to load more and more pills on me—they upped my blood pressure meds, added some potassium, a laxative (because oxycodone often causes constipation) and were making me take a diuretic to get the fluid buildup out of my system faster. It was impossible to take this pileup of pills without something to eat, so I resolved to at least try.

But it was hard to swallow all these pills, especially the potassium pill. It was huge. It reminded me of a horse aspirin I once saw, except it was in a capsule shape. The nurses try to help by breaking the thing in half, but they're still big. I take a magnesium orotate pill at home that's a bit large and I can do it, but at that time in the hospital when I was still sick from all the drugs and not eating, swallowing that thing felt impossible at times.

Speaking of food, I was grateful. There's a lot of homeless or others who don't know where their next meal is going to come from, but here I was having someone come in and offer me meals three times a day. There were even choices I had that I could order ahead of time. I had refused them up till now, but was ready to order this time.

Now, hospital food is bland. They avoid two things most of us crave as if they were pure poison—sugar and salt. I'd been told about the sugar thing from nurse Terry at the pre-op. *Don't have donuts for breakfast and don't drink soda,* she'd told me. Bacteria loves sugar, apparently, and the less sugar in you when you're recovering from major surgery, the faster you'd heal. That seemed persuasive to me.

So when they offered me 7-Up or ginger ale as part of my lunch, it surprised me. Sure, I'll take a ginger ale. The rest of the meal was chicken noodle soup, a yogurt, some crackers and a salad. Well, the ginger ale turned out to be a diet mini can. No surprise, except for the fact that in recent news, they've been talking about how diet sodas can actually cause weight gain even more than regular sodas. The reason is because the chemicals in it that mimic sugar trick your brain into thinking you're ingesting the real stuff, so it releases insulin in anticipation. When insulin levels rise, excess glucose in your bloodstream get stored as body fat. And so on, and so forth. But in this case, weight gain wasn't really an issue. They just didn't want their patients getting sugar. I managed to get though maybe a third of the meal and couldn't take anymore. But I did succeed in getting the pills down.

It was sometime during the fourth day that a different nurse stopped by during the day shift. After going through the routine and asking all the usual questions, she asked me where my heart pillow was. Now, a "heart pillow" in a hospital isn't necessarily the red, heart-shaped kind that looks like a Valentine's adornment. Some hospitals give those out to their heart patients, mine had not. I told her I didn't get one. So she took a regular pillow, folded it in half, and duct-taped the ends together. Now, I had something to hug while sitting up and moving around. I'll talk about the importance of this in the next chapter.

The room I was in was large and separated by three or four draw curtains with a middle section for a nurse's station. On the other side of the room was a man from the Middle East name Ishmael. I came to know details of his situation because of the conversations I heard him having with his main nurse, a tall Japanese man named James with a long, grey ponytail. Like in other situations, I wasn't deliberately eavesdropping; when you're sitting or lying there with nothing else to do, you hear things.

Ishmael had been a smoker since he was a teenager, and he was now 72. Like me, he'd had open-heart surgery, but for a triple coronary bypass. In addition to clogging up his coronary arteries, all those decades of smoking had apparently burned away his cilia, the coating of tiny hairs in the bronchial tubes that wave back and forth spreading mucus which keeps dust and germs and other unwanted things out of the lungs. The result was that for the entire length of my stay, I had to listen to poor Ishmael cough and choke, day and night, in a really bad way. His coughing was the deep down to the bottom of one's lungs kind of coughing. And it came with these horrible gurgling, almost vomiting kind of sounds as his body tried to rid itself of all that stuff he'd inhaled over the years. To help, they gave him one of those "saliva ejector" or "tonsil tip suction" tools that dentists use during a teeth cleaning to suck out the gunk he'd just coughed up. Real fun stuff.

Ishmael was also being a bit ornery with the nurses. He'd make demands that they fix his pillows or adjust the towel over his head or whatever. Sometimes I'd hear him arguing with a nurse about something she was trying to get him to do. But I did have some sympathy. Coughing or sneezing is *painful* after open-heart surgery. Consider the trauma it causes your body to have your sternum sawn in half and held open by a brace for several hours. For the first couple weeks, your entire chest is very delicate and the jerking from coughing produces waves of pain.

The first time I had a small coughing fit, it was so excruciating, I just wanted to pass out. You can feel this defense mechanism somewhere in your brain kick in that does everything it can to stop the next cough. It's intense. And here was poor Ishmael having these constant coughing fits all throughout the day and most of the night, especially when he'd get woken up by something.

Ishmael's recovery must have been more fragile than mine because he wasn't allowed to move by himself. They actually alarmed his chair so that when he tried to get up, the resulting noise would cause staff to rush in and lecture him about the dangers of moving around on his own. This, of course, made him even more irritable.

There was one occasion I won't forget. Ishmael had an adult daughter who came to visit him one evening. She chatted with James for a bit while my nurse did her rounds on me. At some point, Ishmael fell asleep, exhausted from all the commotion and everything that was going on. Later, when the nurses and other staff had left, it was just the three of us in that room separated only by curtains.

I then heard Ishmael's daughter start to cry. It was a soft crying as she tried to muffle it, but I could hear it clearly through the thin curtains. It was one of those moments that gets etched in your mind forever—the cool, quiet, dimly-lit hospital room, the faint beeps and glowing lights from the surrounding equipment, the sound of a daughter weeping for her father. I thought about all the other beds in just our one floor filled with heart patients, their loved ones by their sides wondering what the future held. Many of them, mostly older than me, were in far worse shape and had a much longer road to recovery.

The next image is a rather unflattering photo of my chest one week after surgery. It's quite graphic so don't stare too long if you're squeamish.

Photo: Post surgery incisions

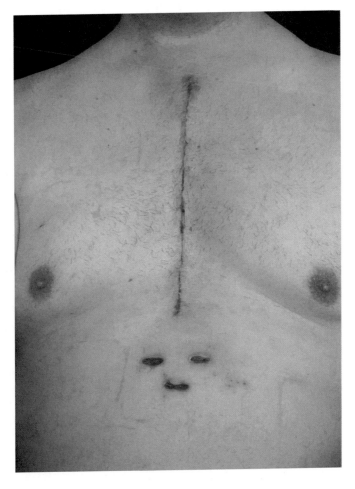

Image source: Kelly Libatique (n.d.). No copyright.

I got the same lecture, or warning really, in terms of the dangers of moving around and accidentally falling. The sternum is a large bone that holds your ribcage together and your heart and lung's main source of protection against impact. The average adult's is maybe 12 inches long. The surgeon used a bone saw to divide it, and now this big bone needs to fuse itself back together. People who've gone through this surgery need to be extra careful those first couple weeks because if you fall and land the wrong way, you'll re-break that bone. The thought was horrifying. I could only start to imagine how painful that would be. Needless to say, I was careful. But for whatever reason, they didn't keep the same eye on me. I'm guessing maybe because, while I was clearly a little despondent, I was very cooperative with the nurses and followed all my instructions. I didn't argue or give anyone a hard time.

At some point between the second and third day, my surgeon, Dr. Dan, came in to check up on me. He was wearing his scrubs and I'm sure had been busy that morning cutting someone else open. He looked and sounded calm and reassuring while he asked questions and told me about my numbers (meaning the daily blood test results for my various levels of potassium, magnesium, phosphate, ionized calcium, white blood cell differential, and a slew of other things). He said I was doing really well and he'd start deciding when various tubes and things could be removed. I told him I couldn't eat the first day and was throwing up and he just nodded and told me it was perfectly normal. A lot of others have it worse with general anesthesia, I was told. I appreciated his visit and wondered how many other patients he did that for each week.

At some point toward the end of the third day, I was told that I was doing so well, they might be removing the drainage tubes under my incision soon. Dr. Dan hadn't lied. That was good, because those things were feeling really uncomfortable, especially when moving.

To give you an idea of what those tubes feel like, think of your solar plexus. It's also called the celiac plexus, but many just say "solar plex." It's called that because it's a mesh of radiating nerve fibers and a network of nerves right there in the middle of your torso. In martial arts or self-defense classes, one of the first things you're taught is how painful it is to strike someone there.

Well, the drainage tubes that are inserted into your body cause a different but similar pain to getting hit in the solar plexus. The tubes reside *behind* the solar plexus and feel like three angry fingers pulling outward from the inside. And they are about as long as the fingers of a person with large hands. It especially hurts when sitting up from a lying position. It's not a lot of fun. So when they told me these were going to get removed, it was good news.

I ate a little dinner on the third day (meaning "Day 2," post-surgery) but not a whole lot. I've had a bad habit my whole life of eating until I feel stuffed, and it was kind of nice that I had no desire to do that. I knew I was losing weight as a result of all this, and I wanted to continue the pattern.

The next morning, after all the blood tests and everything else, I was told that I was doing so well I'd for sure be getting the tubes removed. Now I had more to anticipate. Because of all my pre-surgery research, I'd watched videos of people having these things removed. Nobody liked it. Everyone liked it afterwards, of course, but no one liked having to do it. Like so many things in life. But not because it's painful. That young guy I talked about earlier, the one that was eating on the first day, had said as much. When his tubes were pulled out, he made the comment, "Well, that was unpleasant." So I didn't know what to expect except a lot of, well, unpleasantness.

The individual who removed my tubes was this worker who had a "Surgeon's Assistant" label on his hospital clothes. He was in his mid-30's and looked at you with wide, magnified eyes through thick glasses. He was a nice enough person, but had a kind of robotic, business-like way of going about things. During the course of his day, he inflicted a lot of discomfort or flat-out pain on people as part of many of his duties, but you could tell it didn't phase him. Not that he was insensitive, and I certainly didn't get the impression he was sadistic. He was just immune to not taking personally what had to be some hard feelings from a lot of patients. He spoke in reassuring tones and explained everything that was happening, which I appreciated. But I could understand why having a personality such as his would be a boon with a job like this.

He came in at maybe 10:00 in the morning and asked me if I was ready to have the tubes removed. I just nodded yes while inside I'm yelling *yoo-hoo!* I was glad but also nervous. Using the bed controls, he laid me down flat, then raised the entire bed as high as it would go. He then put on gloves and began pulling out a bunch of pre-packaged items assembled just for this procedure. They included this tube of petroleum jelly like goop, some bandages, small scissors, and other things. He mostly worked in silence, but at one point said this shouldn't hurt, but that it might feel "strange." I didn't bother explaining that I'd seen videos of the procedure done to others already.

He peeled off the large bandage that had covered the three holes in me where the tubes where. It was caked with dried blood. For the first time I saw the holes and the tubes going into my body. It was a weird sight. The tubes were half an inch wide at least in diameter, and the edges of the incisions had been stitched tight to prevent the tubes from sliding. Not a spectacle for the squeamish.

Mr. Surgeon's Assistant began cleaning the area with a wet, disinfectant wipe of some kind. By the way, he did give me his name, but for the life of me I can't remember; one of the many side effects of drugs plus apprehension. He then took some tiny wire-cutting looking scissors and began snipping and then pulling out the stiches around the tubes. After preparing a fresh bandage and getting the goop ready, he placed a cloth over the tube holes and asked me to take a deep breath.

Here we go.

I inhaled as much as I could, and he yanked. I found out later that the holding-the-breath part wasn't for pain, it was actually to prevent air from the tubes going into your body. This is especially important when the tubes go into your lungs like the extra one in my right lung.

When he yanked, the tubes came out quickly, but you can feel them rubbing the edges of the incision holes as they come out from inside your body. And all I can tell you is that it's an inexplicably strange and yes, unpleasant feeling. Fortunately, there aren't pain nerves on the heart or directly around it.

The Surgeon's Assistant stared at me for a moment to gauge my reaction. I think I said, "Well, that felt bizarre."

"I hear that all the time," he said.

As soon as the blood-coated tubes were out, my helper quickly squeezed the petroleum jelly like goop over the three holes and put the new bandage on. I didn't feel immediate relief from the internal pressure the tubes had caused, but I was glad it was over. He started wrapping up the tubes and the other items he'd used for the procedure for disposal. When he picked up the gurgling boxes and moved them to the side next to the wall, it was a great feeling knowing they weren't attached to me anymore.

I looked down at the bandage covering the fourth tube they'd inserted into my right lung. I'd been told that was the "pig-tailed" kind, where the end of it had been bent and fashioned into a little hook. I'd have to wait another day or two for that one to get removed.

Now that I was down to just one tube and one box, I could actually move myself. After some practice I learned how to get out of the bed and transition to the chair without any help. That may not seem like much, but when you've been essentially immobilized for three days, you enjoy that little bit of freedom. I even started taking the initiative to drape an extra gown over my back, pick up my box and exit the room, where I'd do slow laps around the floor. I would run into other heart patients doing the same thing. Most were smiling and seemed to be in a good mood, and I came to understand why. After being in bed, unable to move much and in pain, it felt good to have the freedom to walk on your own. This experience will create in you a sympathy and empathy for those who cannot do simple things like take a little stroll.

It was sometime later that day that the girl with the portable x-ray machine came in again and needed to do another x-ray on me. I was in the chair this time and was surprised to hear that I could just remain where I was during the procedure. As before, the thick, heavy led-filled piece was draped over my lab and all I had to do was sit back. She aimed the big machine at me, which was a good five feet away, and a red lit square with an "X" appeared on my chest again. I was more alert now and it was an odd feeling of being targeted by such a high-tech looking contraption. She hit a button and retreated a few steps back while I heard a soft whir and buzz. Then it was over, thank you for your cooperation. She wheeled the machine out of the room. Amazing. I remember the days when they had to wheel your whole bed to the x-ray room and place you under this giant, stationary mechanism.

Day number five (or day four if you don't count surgery day) was the day the "pig tailed" tube in my right lung was removed. My surgeon's assistant friend with the glasses was there again to do the job. He told me that it would be pretty much the exact same thing as when the first three tubes were removed, but for some reason I wasn't so sure. We went through the same process. I waited patiently while he broke out his stuff. The only difference this time was that I remained in a semi-seated position on the bed.

After the bandage and stitches were removed, and we were ready, he pressed a cloth over the incision and told me to take a big breath. I did, felt a yank, and then experienced a horrible, startling pain as the little "pigtail" of the hose hooked the inside of my skin as it was coming out. Seriously, it hurt.

I grimaced and then my jaw dropped as I let out some kind of groan/sigh combination and said, "Ooohh… that…hurt."

The Surgeon's Assistant just looked at me for a moment with those big eyes of his and then continued. Again, I didn't get the impression that he didn't care, he just went on with the job he had to do. Pain and discomfort were simply a part of that. I was a bit surprised though as to how quickly he'd tugged. He knew all about these hoses with the little hooks so he should have used a different technique, in my opinion. But then what did I know. I do know if I ever go through something like that again, I will voice my concerns before the yanking.

My surgery had been on a Monday morning and it was now Thursday. My gown was filthy with sweat and blood stains and I'd not had a shower since very early Monday morning. I was really glad I'd shaved clean because my normal beard would have been uncomfortably long by now.

There were still a couple things hanging out of my body: the wires that they could use to zap and jump start me. These, like the tubes, were actually embedded in my chest and went up to my heart. I didn't really feel them when moving around, or maybe I did, but they were so small in comparison to the drain tubes.

The second thing were the four or five EKG electrode stickers that were mostly congregated on one side. I didn't even feel them, but they were connected to that annoying box that I carried around in my gown pocket. The nurses had come in a couple times and changed the batteries on it by now, and I was getting tired of carrying it around. If I continued to improve and my numbers looked good, I could get that stuff off and maybe be released tomorrow, I was told.

Friday morning came and I got through more than half my breakfast. The bland egg-whites omelet was getting old, but the yogurt still tasted good. I swallowed most of my pills but snuck the ginormous potassium pills into the garbage after wrapping them in a napkin. I just couldn't get them down.

The nurse who started the 8:00 AM shift came in and after doing her routine, told me it looked like I was going to let go today? Really? Wow. Some people spend weeks in the hospital after open-heart surgery. It appeared that my roommate Ishmael would be doing that. I'd just been cut open on Monday and here it was only Friday.

Dr. Dan came in around maybe 10:00 AM and told me once again my numbers were doing great. Later, the nurse practitioner paid a visit and told me I was one of their "superstars" for how quickly I was recovering. I was still deep in the woods, but improving fast. She was going to call my wife and see if I could be picked up that afternoon. I had thought for sure I'd not be able to go home until at least Saturday or Sunday and was now wondering if my wife would be available.

The time finally came for those two wires attached to my heart to be removed. My surgeon's assistant friend came in to pay me one last visit. I watched him warily as he broke out his gear. This time the procedure wasn't quite as complicated in terms of the stuff needed.

He raised my bed as usual and after getting prepped, I was told to hold my breath once again. I obediently did as instructed, and then he started pulling. This actually hurt a lot more than when the first three big tubes were yanked out of my abdomen, but not as much as the pigtailed tube. The best way I can describe it is little rope burns at each of the two holes. These holes were significantly smaller, but as the wires were removed, they burned and stung something awful against the edges of the wounds. Fortunately, the pain didn't last as they aren't that long. It's just another one of those icky, weird feelings you never want to voluntarily experience again.

Now that those were out, I only had the four or five electrode stickers for my little portable EKG device, and the IV that had been in my right arm since Monday morning.

A nurse came in at some point with a small basin of warm, soapy water and a sponge. It occurred to me again that I'd not bathed since Monday. I had looked at the dried blood stains on my gown and wondered how filthy it was with sweat and everything else, but what could I do? She was in her 50's with a calm, gentle smile. I'd been told by others in their video-documented experiences that when offered a sponge bath by the nurses, take it. Even though it looked like I was actually getting out later that day, I decided to just do it so I'd feel better.

The nurse, obviously very practiced, carefully put a towel over my privates and then lifted the old, soiled gown over my head. She then gave me a sponge to wipe down my arms and front while she wiped down my back. After lying on that bed for a week, the warm, soapy water felt absolutely wonderful. Afterwards I was given a brand new, clean gown and felt quite refreshed.

I don't remember how much time had passed, not even an hour, when another nurse came in and pealed the EKG electrode stickers off. This process always pulls away several chest hairs (for us guys anyway) but that was nothing compared to what I'd been through the last several days. Besides, this was the fourth time I'd had those stickers taken off me. What was a relief though was when they finally hauled that EKG device away and I no longer had to carry it around in my flimsy hospital gown pocket. I was really starting to get free.

The 8:00 AM shift nurse came in shortly before lunch and told me my wife had been contacted and was on her way. They'd be bringing my clothes to me so I could put back on what I'd worn on Monday morning. Wow, was I being blessed.

Someone from food services came in and asked if I was going to be needing lunch. I proudly told her that I didn't need it because I was getting released. She smiled at my good news and left, but I'd regret this decision as there was still a bit of waiting to do. Nothing moves quickly in hospitals unless it's a life or death emergency.

Close to noon, my wife came in and the reality that I was going to be getting out of there was becoming, well, a reality. We tried to hug but my chest felt too delicate.

Someone brought in a plastic bag with the clothes I wore in on Monday morning—the ragged jogging pants, t-shirt and jacket. I changed as quickly as I could but still had to move slowly because of the huge incision and three gaping holes on my chest. Bending over was a problem in particular, and after sitting in the chair, I had to ask my wife to remove the hospital no-slip socks and put my own back on. When I stood up, fully dressed for the first time in five days, it felt really good.

At some point while I was changing, I had my first coughing fit. I felt it coming and tried to stop it, but couldn't. I held a pillow close to my chest while the first cough came. I hurt so bad, I had to sit down. Then a second and a third cough came. I was wincing grimacing and wondering how my roommate Ishmael had managed. Finally it stopped. I stood up again to finished changing as fast as I could.

But all my rushing was for naught because I still had the IV stuck in and taped to my arm and I had to wait for a nurse to remove it. The nurse was making her rounds and nowhere to be found. I stared at it, tempting myself to just do it. I could have used the intercom to call someone, but decided to give it a few before bugging them.

Twenty minutes later or so she did return and that little needle and tape job on the crook of my arm was finally removed. My wife went down to get the car and have it waiting for me in the pick-up lane while a wheelchair was called. Similar to the day I got my angiogram, a "volunteer" was going to wheel me downstairs. I waited as patiently as I could.

Finally, a lady in her late 50's with a pleasant smile and a thick Russian accent came to get me. We rode most of the way in silence which I appreciated. When the hospital entrance doors opened and I felt the cool San Francisco air rush in and hit me, it was most satisfying. I pointed out our car and was wheeled up to it. I carefully got myself into the back seat and my wife buckled me in, following the instructions to put a pillow between my chest and the seatbelt.

We drove away, homeward bound at last.

Recovery at Home

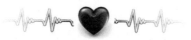

**"It does not matter how slowly you go
along as long as you don't stop."**

—Confucius

In just five days after getting my chest sawed open, I was back at home. And so began a strange next 30 days or so.

Bear in mind that many people who undergo this kind of surgery are in the hospital for much longer. I was still definitely in full-on recovery mode. Although being at home made it seem like everything was "okay now," it was not, and that became apparent right away.

They want to know who is going to be helping you at home and if that person will be there full time for the first few days. They, meaning your care staff. Among others, mine included my cardiologist as well as Joanne, the nurse practitioner who had spoken to me during the pre-op. For some this might be easy to arrange, for others, not so much. But believe me when I say you *will* need help with even the smallest of things.

First off, I was still in the danger zone of rebreaking my sternum. The thought was overwhelming. If I tripped and fell on something like a chair or a table edge, or if I stumbled and instinctively held out one or both of my arms to brace the fall…Wow, I could end up getting rushed to emergency, then back to the operating table.

Next, as I mentioned before, I was cold. My circulation was off, and I was on three times the blood pressure meds I'd been on before surgery (this dosage would be reduced in time). This had brought my pulse down, and even with the temperature inside the house above 70, I felt like I needed a thick jacket, gloves, and a beanie cap. I still look at pictures of me dressed like I'm on a snow outing, but I'm just on the couch snuggling with my dog.

I set up a sort of "station" at the corner of the main living room couch. Next to me was a small table, on which I had bottles of water, a Kleenex box, my pill bottles, and so on. I was content to stay there at my post for most of the first few days, not wanting to move except to do some easy walking exercises. This little spot would become very important because for the first several weeks at home, between your walking routines, you'll mostly be sitting or lying down sleeping.

The first time I ventured outside with my wife, we slowly made our way up the sidewalk to the local park, and then did one slow lap. I shuffled along like a 90-year-old. It's a small park, but one full lap felt like a victory. I was tired and feeling a little dizzy and I remember staring at the sidewalk edge as we walked. One of the things that recovering from heart surgery does is that it makes you aware of certain dangers you never thought about before. A sidewalk curb is only what, six inches? But as I'm walking, I'm looking at the edge and shuddering at the just the thought of accidentally stepping off and falling forward on the hard asphalt. The idea was terrifying.

One of the information pamphlets I was given during the pre-op was this illustrated series on how _not_ to use your arms and elbows in ways we all normally do. Example, when sitting in or standing up from a chair, you cannot use your arms or elbows on the arm rests. You must use leg power only. When you open your arms and put weight or any kind of pressure on them, it creates just the kind of pulling outward and "apart" tension on your sternum you need to avoid.

You also can't pick up heavy objects. I've always been pretty physically strong and did a lot of weight training in my younger years. But after surgery, you cannot lift things that puts stress your chest area. That means no lifting, especially with just one arm. You can pick up smaller things using both arms and keeping the object close to your body, but nothing else.

But the hardest movement with regards to avoiding arms and elbows was getting in and out of bed. This takes practice, and I suggest you or your loved one rehearse this prior to surgery. First, get a pillow and hug it close to your chest. This will remind you not to accidentally reach out to brace yourself. Next, you must sit as deep up on the bed as possible. Now raise your feet off the ground and allow gravity to slowly pull you down while turning and sort of rolling on to the bed.

I learned right away that getting into the right position before rolling on to the bed was important. The reason is that once you've lain down, it's not easy to adjust yourself. Say you were too high up, and your head was hitting the backrest, or you were too close to the side and felt like you were going to fall off. Before surgery, you don't even think about making these little adjustments to settle in. But when your sternum is trying to heal and you're unable to use your arms, it's not easy. As well, the muscles in your chest produce stinging, burning pains when flexed for any reason. Even some of the smallest movements like reaching up to adjust the pillow seemed impossible.

Getting back out of bed is even more difficult. This is why I did a lot of sit-ups before surgery—you need a strong core. With a pillow hugged firmly to your chest, you must turn your body and ease up into a sitting position. It helps to let your feet dangle over the side first. It's harder than you might think. Give it a try and you'll know what I mean.

To ease the struggle of getting in and out of bed, I slept without covers for almost a month. This was November so it was chilly. I'd lay out a jacket or a couple of flannel shirts or sweatshirts to the side of where I was going to be lying. Then after getting into a position where I thought I could sleep, I'd drag the shirts over me to act as blankets. That way, in the morning, I wouldn't have to add the struggle of getting out of thick, heavy covers. Mornings, by the way, are the most painful because the drugs have worn off throughout the night.

My bed is a little high off the ground, at waist level. This made it more difficult. There was one scare I'll never forget. The floor in my bedroom is hardwood which makes it slippery when wearing socks. I was getting out of bed and when my feet hit the floor, they slid backwards. I had to catch and brace myself against the bed with my elbows to keep from sliding all the way back and send me crashing to the floor. It was frightening and it hurt; I could feel the strain on my sternum. Fortunately, nothing happened beyond the pain and the scare.

After the first three or four weeks of having such a hard time with the bed, we ordered a nice La-Z-Boy chair, the kind where you push a button and the back goes down as the foot rest comes up. We should have done this much sooner and would have, had we known how difficult it was going to be for me to get in and out of bed. That chair became a lifesaver. If you have the room for one of these and you're getting ready for heart surgery, get one. I spent many long hours napping during the day and sleeping at night at times as it was so much easier to get in and out of it.

Speaking of pain, I was warned about chest muscle pain. While I didn't feel a lot of it in a consistent way, I did feel it at times with certain movements, like when I was lying down or sitting up. I think it's because as I was hugging the pillow and sitting up, I instinctively flexed my chest muscles. The pains were these piercing waves that dance back and force, like an electrical current going through nerves in your chest. They aren't fun, but at least they weren't a nagging, ongoing thing.

Speaking of chest muscles, I lost almost all strength. It kind of scared me. I'm not some athlete or body builder, but before surgery I was doing light weight resistance training, long walks, and lots of pushups. I could easily put my feet up on a chair and do 30 or 40 elevated pushups.

Well, while waiting for your sternum to re-fuse, just the *idea* of getting on the ground and doing pushups was fear-provoking. In fact, for the first month, I'd have been afraid to get down on the ground for anything, for fear I would not be able to get back up. It's hard, after all, to get off the ground using just your legs. But I think it was toward the end of the third month I decided I'd try some pushups again. I carefully got down to the floor and slowly put weight on my arms, one at a time, making sure I didn't feel any alarming pain. I did not. So I straightened out my legs, lifted my knees of the ground, and went down for a pushup. To my shock, I didn't have the strength to come back up—not even for one pushup. It was an awful feeling. To get off the floor again, I had to roll over, sit up and do it one knee at a time.

It took months to get any chest strength back, and almost a year later, I still don't have the strength I used to. Admittedly though, I've not been working that hard at it. Physical activity in general will diminish and stay that way unless you make very proactive efforts to get back into it.

Photo: Dressed for winter and bundled up at my "station"

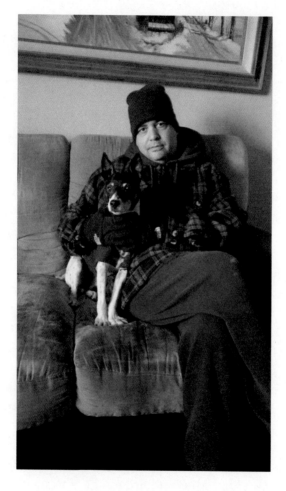

Image source: Kelly Libatique (n.d.). No copyright.

In the beginning, I had a home nurse come see me for a total of six visits, once a week. It was kind of comforting to have a medical professional see you when you don't feel like going anywhere like a crowded doctor's office. She was a young woman from Spain named Maria and had a thick accent. She was instrumental in encouraging me not to be cynical about having to take Coumadin for the rest of my life.

"I hate this stupid drug," I would grumble.

"Don't say that," she would say. She went on to tell me how good it was that this drug was available to people in my position.

Maria always came with a portable INR (international normalized ratio) tester device and would poke my finger and put a drop of blood on this flat plastic piece inserted into the end of the little machine. After a few seconds, it would read how quickly my blood was coagulating. She also checked my wounds to ensure they were healing properly, checked my blood pressure, and listened to my heart. After the six visits, she said I was doing so well she was officially "discharging" me and no longer had to come by. That meant I had to start going to the hospital lab for more INR tests, and I've been doing that ever since.

Speaking of INR, I was also assigned to some individuals from the hospital's "Coumadin Office." They do one thing: help manage people who take this drug. It's great they exist because earlier I mentioned my grandmother who took too much of the stuff and almost bled to death. On the other hand, it's astonishing that there are so many people who take it for whatever reason(s). Is it our diets or lifestyle? Nurse Maria would send them the results of my INR tests and then they'd make recommendations on what my daily dose should be. They still do that for me now after almost a year; the hospital lab now sends the results. The difference is that instead of once a week, I am doing a test every 30 to 40 days now.

After a month I was doing two, then eventually three laps around the park. My cardiologist was so proud of me. And you do feel victorious. If there is one piece of advice I would give to anyone going through this—get up and walk as much as you can. Starting on day of your surgery. Push yourself. You must force yourself to do it as much as possible. This is key to a quick recovery.

Getting in and out of bed normally and without pain came at about the third month. By then, I was spending most nights back in my bed which made sleep better because that's where my CPAP setup is. The first time I sat up without pain was a milestone.

I would say that somewhere between the fifth and sixth month, I was pretty much feeling normal. I look a little different—there's a big, permanent scar that runs the length of my sternum. The sternum wires underneath don't show on the outside, but are a permanent accessory in my body, unless they cause problems. I've heard they can be removed fairly easily, but it requires going under general anesthesia again, something I don't want to do. But I would if necessary.

You might be asking, what permanent changes in my body have I felt since surgery? Well, a couple things. First, my heartbeat is louder and I can really feel it thumping more in my chest. The reason is that the heart muscle has a tight covering that surrounds it, a lining sac called the *pericardium*. To get to your heart, surgeons must cut this open.

I'm told it kind of resembles tightly wrapped cellophane and when sliced, the edges quickly shrink back.

In the old days, meaning when heart surgery was new, they attempted to pull the edges of the pericardium back into place and sew them together. But they found it didn't work and hindered the heart's beating. So nowadays, they leave this sac open and there it remains in your body like that. The result is that you no longer have a cushion or layer between your heart and the sternum bone and so your heart both sounds louder and feels like it's beating stronger. It's a strange sensation. I do voice-over on the side and use a very sensitive large diaphragm condenser microphone. When I'm really quiet, I can hear my heartbeat going through it to the recording.

Then there's the mechanical aortic valve. This thing has a subtle tick-tick to it. Not like a clock's tick, more like if you made a soft *tst-tst* sound with your tongue. It's hard to explain. But there are many moments throughout the day when I can hear this faint tick in my ear, especially at night when going to sleep. I've had people near me tell me they can hear the tick as well. I tell people, *I'm a real-life cyborg and a walking, talking Timex watch now.* And it's kind of true.

How about being on Coumadin/Warfarin? Well, after almost a year of being on this drug, I've no major side effects. I still don't relish the idea of having to take it for the rest of my life, but hey, I'm alive. If you've heard it will cause you to bruise easier, you heard right. If I bump into something or even if I'm unscrewing a really tight lid and I have to squeeze it really hard, I'll see bruise marks on my skin. If I sit in a chair too long with one ankle resting on my knee for a long time, I will sometimes get a bruise where my ankle was for a few days.

In regard to keeping my INR level between the prescribed 2 and 3, that's not been difficult. Other kinds of surgery or conditions require more precise windows. My cardiologist told me that because of where my valve is, at the aortic root position, there's a lot of pressure there so clotting is less likely than in other places of the body. But generally speaking, what a window between 2 and 3 means is that if a person not on this drug gets a cut, their blood will start clotting within about nine seconds. But mine won't start clotting until between 21 and 23 seconds. I've already discussed the implications of this. Too much of the drug and the next you know, you've got internal bleeding that won't stop. Too little and my mechanical valve can start clotting up. I don't like it, but again, I'm alive and my life really hasn't change significantly because of it.

My surgeon, Dr. Dan, told me about this young guy, not even 30, who needed a valve replaced. But because he was a hardcore skier, he insisted on a biological tissue valve (I don't remember if it was a pig's or a cow's) because he didn't want to be on Coumadin and worry every time he fell or got injured. Dr. Dan is worried for him because he believes it won't be long before the valve fails and Mr. Skier will be back on the operating table. For me, being at the age of 49 and not athletic to begin with, the decision to go with the mechanical valve was easier.

Final Thoughts

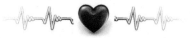

**"Tell me and I forget.
Teach me and I remember.
Involve me and I learn."**

—Benjamin Franklin

And so, as I approach my one-year anniversary since surgery, I come to the end of this narrative. If you or someone you know is facing a similar situation, and you're reading this as part of your preparation, I hope I've helped shed some light on what is to come. Maybe you're just curious. Whatever the reason, here are some conclusions I've drawn.

Life is not just precious, it's astonishing. We've all heard how valuable life is, still though, the tendency is to take what you've got for granted, especially when it comes to health. Not just yourself and your abilities, but the people around you. But when you have an experience like this, one that forces you to wave your hand over the flames of death, as it were, you see things in a different light.

I've seen my heart beating on a screen, the little flaps of my valves opening and closing. I've heard the swishing and swirling of blood passing through valves and arteries. And now, especially in quiet moments when I'm meditating or lying in bed and I can feel my pulse, I have a whole new appreciation of the ingenious and intricate design that comes together to keep our bodies alive.

I have a few lessons learned I'd like to share. The first is to take charge of your health and be proactive. As early as in my 20's, I'd been warned I had both blood pressure and sleeping problems. The younger me figured I could control these things with lifestyle, eating right, managing my weight and so on. I wouldn't even learn the term "sleep apnea" until much later. But both conditions were quite serious. The result of my procrastination was permanent damage to my body that later needed fixing.

I don't know why I waited so long. Fear? Pride? Whatever the case, my advice to you is, suck it up and go to the doctor's. I may not have been able to prevent my aortic aneurism, but if my apnea had been treated sooner, I certainly would have enjoyed, especially my 30's decade, a lot more, as I would have had much better sleep. Life is short and we have technology today that can help. Utilize it.

And don't forget me having to fill in cavities on my two remaining wisdom teeth right before surgery. It wasn't that it was such a bad experience, it was just one more stressor on the table. Twenty years ago, I could have taken the dentist's advice and prevented all that by going to the oral surgeon and having those teeth removed. But no…I waited. Actually, I just pretended the problem didn't exist. Lot of good that did.

The one thing I'll give myself a get-out-of-jail-free card for is the bicuspid disease I was born with. Obviously, there was nothing I could have done to prevent this. This disease affects only 1.3% of adults and is twice as likely to affect men than women. And statistically, I was quite typical as

this condition tends to rear its ugly head and start causing problems between a person's fourth and fifth decade
in life. Did my blood pressure and sleep apnea contribute
to a faster deterioration of my aortic valve? It's uncertain,
but my surgeon is pretty sure the severity of the aneurysm
contributed. Doesn't matter now. What's important is that
the whole thing was caught in time to save my life.

How about emotions and reactions? I've always had
a problem with reacting to the ugly behavior of certain
people. Case in point, I live in the San Francisco East Bay
area. I don't know how things are where you live, but here
everyone is in an insanely mad rush. Particularly in the
last several years, the freeways have become Germany's
autobahn, and speed limits mean nothing anymore. You
could be doing 25 mph over the limit in the right most
lane and people are still barreling past you or bullying you
out of the way by tailgating and flashing their brights. This
is standard operating procedure at most times of the day
anymore. I used to react badly to this kind of thing, I'd
fume and feel my heart rate and blood pressure shoot up.
Sometimes I'd respond in ways I'm not proud of.

But since surgery, I've tried to take it easier. It's not
worth it. Let other people rush to their graves, you don't
have to react to them. The tendency I have to cling to a
thought or feeling that bothers me is still a weakness, but
I have a different perspective on things now. Why should I
let others control my emotions? When I'm tempted to stew
on something until it angers or frustrates me, I breath deep,
slow down, and find something positive to distract myself
with. To mitigate reactions like this, you need to be deliberate and put them out of your mind. I imagine wadding them
up like a virtual piece of paper and throwing them into a

virtual garbage can. It takes training and practice to do this, and it's not easy at first because you're resting engrained habits. I still slip now and then, but I'm doing better.

Regarding pessimism and negativity...I consciously peppered this writing with a lot of the cynical thoughts and dark humor I was experiencing at the time of my diagnosis and on through the tests and preparation for surgery. Not to glorify it, but to be honest in what I was feeling. I humbly admit I focused on the things that could go wrong. It took many years of hard, habit-forming work to become that way.

But this whole experience has changed me quite a bit. For example, my general distrust of people has changed. To get through something like open-heart surgery, I had to become totally vulnerable and rely on the help from a lot of people. At any time, I could have been mistreated or taken advantage of, but no one did. A few showed that I was clearly *just another patient*, but no one was callous or acted like I was a burden. For the most part, I was met with kindness, generosity, compassion and sympathy, from total strangers no less. I had to place not just my trust, but my actual life in the hands of others, and that did something to me.

Then there's independence and having control. When I say control, I'm not talking about controlling others. In fact, I don't like people who control others via guilt, manipulation, intimidation, or scheming. That stuff really bothers me. I'm talking about being in control of one's own destiny and circumstances. Open-heart surgery will remove any illusions you have of control. You start to appreciate the little things and understand that every beat of your heart and every breath of air you take is a borrowed gift that could be taken away at any time. That's not to be morbid or anything, it's actually an encouragement to just stop and take the time to appreciate the moments of each day. When someone else has to help you use the bathroom, take a shower, or put on your socks, you get humbled quickly. It will change your perspective on those that are stuck in bed or have to live permanently with certain disabilities.

I mentioned I've had a hard time trusting others. Not that I go around paranoid with a victim's mentality or persecution complex. I just have always thought most people do what they do to serve their own self-interests and don't really care about most others. Terrible way to think, I know. But looking back at all the people who came in and out of my life in the months leading up to surgery and then the months afterwards, I realized there are more good people in the world than I'd thought. There were so many who went out of their way to either be encouraging, be of extra service, or just plain be nice. They didn't have to.

In all walks of life there are those who are naturally more friendly and better at connecting than others. I happen to be one of those that isn't so good at making connections, so I really appreciated it when people went that extra mile on my behalf. They weren't going to get paid any more to smile or be pleasant, they just did it. In my ripe, middle age, a lot of these people, many of whom were younger than me, taught this old dog some new tricks.

I've never felt particularly entitled to special treatment, but if you're that kind of person, get ready to be humbled. When a nurse tells you it's going to be a few minutes because someone else needs their attention, just remember that when your time comes, another will be waiting on you. You're surrounded by people who are in the same or similar situation as you. Their lives have been every bit as disrupted and inconvenienced as yours. Like you, they'd rather be anywhere else than stuck in a bed with needles and tubes in their bodies. They have family and friends they'd rather be with. They have dogs and cats back home that are anxiously awaiting the return of their master. Are you more exclusive than they are? No. While we all should be treated with dignity and respect, we should all get it equally.

Another lesson: prepare your home beforehand. I'll start with slip-on shoes. If you don't have a pair, get one before your surgery. The act of bending down and struggling with footwear is going be impossible. When you shower, make sure your towels and clean clothes are at a comfortable arm height and won't require any kind of reaching effort to get to them. This includes anything you have to get to throughout the day, like food, water, your pill bottles, etcetera. Have the person you live with arrange things like this for you.

Photo: Slip-On house shoes

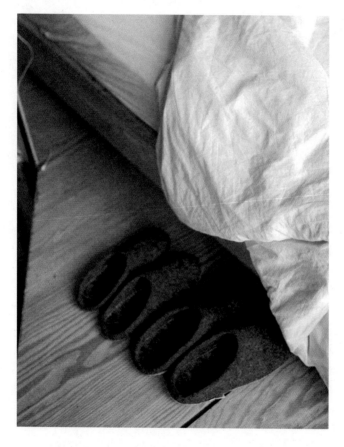

Photo by Anna Maiwald on Unsplash (Aug 17, 2020).
Retrieved from https://unsplash.com/photos/f2SFqYVXlFI

I've also learned something about patience. In addition to being patient with hospital staff and people you live with, you've absolutely got to be patient with yourself. You're going to be useless for a few weeks—deal with it. The stuff on top of your refrigerator or in the kitchen cabinets that you easily grabbed before are going to seem hopelessly out of reach. Your dog will be expecting that daily walk, but you just won't be able to for awhile. If you drop something on the floor, you may not be able to get it.

Now you may think, oh that's cool, I don't mind taking a break from life. Well, think again. If you're an independent person like myself, this can be excruciatingly frustrating. It's one thing to feel lazy and want a respite, it's quite another to be physically incapable of performing simple tasks you'd not given a second thought to before all this. Besides, you're going to be bored at home. You'll reach a point where you've re-watched your favorite movies and read a few books and you'll want more to do. You'll want to be useful, but you won't be able to.

I'll throw in one last out-of-the-way blurb. Shortly before getting ready to publish this, it came out that Arnold Schwarzenegger had a second heart valve replaced. The first time it was his pulmonary valve in 2018, this time his aortic valve, like mine. You may not like him or his politics, but at age 73, he just might be an inspiration for you. I grew up with the first Terminator movie, so news about the former California governor often piques my interest. I'd heard that his pulmonary valve was replaced by a human donor; I guess when you're rich and famous, that's an option. It's been rumored he damaged his heart from steroid use when he was young and in competition. Another lesson to be learned for all of us.

I'll end this by saying I decided to document my journey after sharing a few things on YouTube posts related to surgery or recovery. I had a lot of people who were facing similar situations ask me for advice. Some were quite frightened, as I had been, others just wanted to know what to expect. After detailing some of what I'd been through, I thought, why not just put it all down for whoever to read at any time?

If you're one of those facing open-heart surgery like I was, be grateful for the day in age in which we live. If you were a heart patient back in the 1950's, this would all be new and experimental. Many of those people died because the technology and knowhow just wasn't there yet. But today, this kind of thing has been done tens of thousands of times around the world and the knowledge is there to give you the best odds possible.

Your journey won't be tearless. But what you'll encounter are hundreds of people who've chosen the medical profession as their career because they genuinely care about the healing and comfort of others. For someone like me, that was a pleasant surprise. If I can get through it, so can you.

Take care and God bless.

Made in the USA
Monee, IL
20 July 2022